KETOGE

THE COMPLETE KETOGENIC DIET MEAL PLAN RECIPE GUIDE FOR BEGINNERS

By K. Connors

© **Copyright 2017 By K. Connors - All Rights Reserved.**

Copyright © 2017 *Ketogenic Diet.* All rights reserved. No part of this publication may be reproduced, distributed, or transmitted in any form or by any means, including photocopying, recording, or other electronic or mechanical methods, without the prior written permission of the publisher, except in the case of brief quotations embodied in critical reviews and certain other noncommercial uses permitted by copyright law. This also includes conveying via e-mail without permission in writing from the publisher. All information within this book is of relevant content and written solely for motivation and direction. No financial guarantees. All information is considered valid and factual to the writer's knowledge. The author is not associated or affiliated with any company or brand mentioned in the book, therefore does not purposefully advertise nor receives payment for doing so.

Table of Contents

Introduction 12

Mayonnaise Cream 15

   Ingredients: 15

   Directions: 16

Classic Keto Cornbread... 17

   Ingredients: 17

   Directions: 18

Zesty Blueberry Cake.. 19

   Ingredients: 19

   Directions: 20

Blue Summer Mojito Pops 21

   Ingredients: 21

   Directions: 22

Cheesy Cherries Frittata 23

   Ingredients: 24

   Directions: 24

Meaty Pepper Popper Nachos 25

   Ingredients: 25

   Directions: 26

Fall's Meatloaf Cups 27

   Ingredients: 27

Directions: 28

Herbed Crispy Chicken Thighs 29

   Ingredients: 30

   Directions: 30

Beef Zoodles Ragu 31

   Ingredients: 31

   Directions: 32

Golden Chicken Thighs with Cream Sauce 33

   Ingredients: 33

   Directions: 34

Seared Steak with Keto Butter Sauce 35

   Ingredients: 35

   Directions: 36

Sunny Chicken Cream Skillet 37

   Ingredients: 37

   Directions: 38

Salisbury Steak Patties with Mushroom Gravy 40

   Ingredients: 40

   Directions: 41

Shrimp Zoodles Sauté 43

   Ingredients: 43

   Directions: 44

Seared Cajun Salmon 45
    Ingredients: 46
    Directions: 46
Roasted Shrimp and Asparagus 47
    Ingredients: 47
    Directions: 48
Nutty Chicken and Broccoli Stir Fry 49
    Ingredients: 50
    Directions: 50
Creamy Cauliflower Chowder 51
    Ingredients: 51
    Directions: 52
Seasoned Cod Skillet 53
    Ingredients: 54
    Directions: 54
Meatballs Wedding Soup 55
    Ingredients: 55
    Directions: 56
Creamy Keto Alfredo 58
    Ingredients: 58
    Directions: 59
Cheesy and Saucy Chicken Breasts 60

Ingredients: 60

Directions: 61

Rosemary Cloud Flat Buns 63

Ingredients: 63

Directions: 64

Herbed Tri-Tip 65

Ingredients: 65

Directions: 66

Black Forest Stuffed Chicken Breasts 67

Ingredients: 67

Directions: 68

Glazed Teriyaki Skewers 69

Ingredients: 70

Directions: 70

Spiralized Bacon Soup 71

Ingredients: 71

Directions: 72

Glazed Shrimp Skewers 73

Ingredients: 73

Directions: 74

Grilled Rosy Chops 75

Ingredients: 75

Directions:	76
Macadamia and Chocolate Bombs	77
Ingredients:	77
Directions:	78
Juicy Ropa Vija	79
Ingredients:	79
Directions:	80
Seared Steak with Mushroom	81
Ingredients:	81
Directions:	82
Fancy Stuffed Beef Heart	83
Ingredients:	83
Directions:	84
Orangy Steak Kebab	86
Ingredients:	86
Directions:	87
Chocolate Chip Cookies	88
Ingredients:	88
Directions:	89
Cheesy Cornbread Bacon	91
Ingredients:	91
Directions:	92

Melted Sandwich 93
    Ingredients: 93
    Directions: 94

Golden Cheese Gratin 96
    Ingredients: 96
    Directions: 97

Spring Muffins 98
    Ingredients: 98
    Directions: 99

Tamari Steak Satay 101
    Ingredients: 101
    Directions: 102

Meaty Rainbow Stir Fry 103
    Ingredients: 103
    Directions: 104

Minty Wild Sea Bass 105
    Ingredients: 105
    Directions: 106

Sweet and Sour Apple Meatballs 107
    Ingredients: 107
    Directions: 108

Grammy Hassel-back Chicken Winner 110

Ingredients: 110

Directions: 111

Shredded River Roast 112

Ingredients: 112

Directions: 113

Tasty Lunch Rush Skillet 114

Ingredients: 114

Directions: 115

Creamy Bacon Carbonara 116

Ingredients: 116

Directions: 117

Love on a Plate 118

Ingredients: 118

Directions: 119

Frank's Hot Buffalo Casserole 121

Ingredients: 121

Directions: 122

Italian Style Pepperoni Pizza 124

Ingredients: 124

Directions: 125

Nutty Chicken Bites 126

Ingredients: 126

Directions: 127

Chicken Rolls Soup 128

    Ingredients: 128

    Directions: 129

Crispy Parmesan Nuggets 130

    Ingredients: 130

    Directions: 131

Parmesan Sea Knight 132

    Ingredients: 132

    Directions: 133

Tipsy Chicken Picatta 134

    Ingredients: 135

    Directions: 135

Macadamia Snap Cookies 137

    Ingredients: 137

    Directions: 138

Salmon fritters 139

    Ingredients: 139

    Directions: 140

Festive Turkey Breast Roast 141

    Ingredients: 141

    Directions: 142

Tanned Pumpkin Toast 143

    Ingredients: 143

    Directions: 144

Restaurant Style Lobster Chowder 146

    Ingredients: 146

    Directions: 147

Conclusion 148

Introduction

Embracing the keto diet has never been and will never be easier than now! The times where you had to spend hours online searching for recipes and wondering if those recipes were actually tasty or healthy enough are long gone. To save you some time, we have combined 60 of the easiest and tastiest keto recipes ever, all in one book that will change your life.

It is no secret now that being on a diet is almost like a trend, but against the judgment of many, it is not a celebrity thing. It is without a doubt a very efficient way to actually lose weight in a short span of time while staying healthy. The keto diet is the right path for you to get that body you always desired and fit into that dress or suit you always dreamed of. In addition to becoming healthy and having a killer body, what you might not know is that the keto diet is not only about weight loss; it has many other benefits that are beneficial to your body by getting rid of those unwanted toxins lurking inside. Some of these benefits are:

Significant weight reduction:

I am one of those individuals that must be munching on something more often than not. I get ravenous after a brief span of eating. If you resemble me, you definitely realize that this craving is the fundamental reason for putting on weight. Recently, some individuals have endeavored to eat less or to take meds to kill their cravings, which badly effect their internal bodily functions. With the keto diet, you consume less calories, so you don't need to stress over significant weight gain. Low carb sustenance has a tendency to effectively top you off and reduce your undying want to eat more, which means you won't feel hungry all the time any longer.

Decrease the destructive fat:

We have distinctive fats in our body. However, a standout amongst the most hurtful of them is a destructive fat that tends to wrap around the organs. This may drive aggravation, insulin resistance, and different illnesses. This is how the keto diet slims you down and is genuinely helpful in light of the fact that it diminishes that fat and consequently decreases the probability of you having an illness.

Builds the great cholesterol:

There are two sorts of cholesterols, the awful one is called LDL and it diverts the fat from the liver towards alternate parts of the body. This makes you put on weight. Then, there is the great cholesterol which is called HDL and it does the inverse, conveying the cholesterol towards the liver where it can be applied or reused.

The keto eating routine helps increment this great cholesterol which implies weight reduction for you and additionally lowers the danger of you developing a coronary illness.

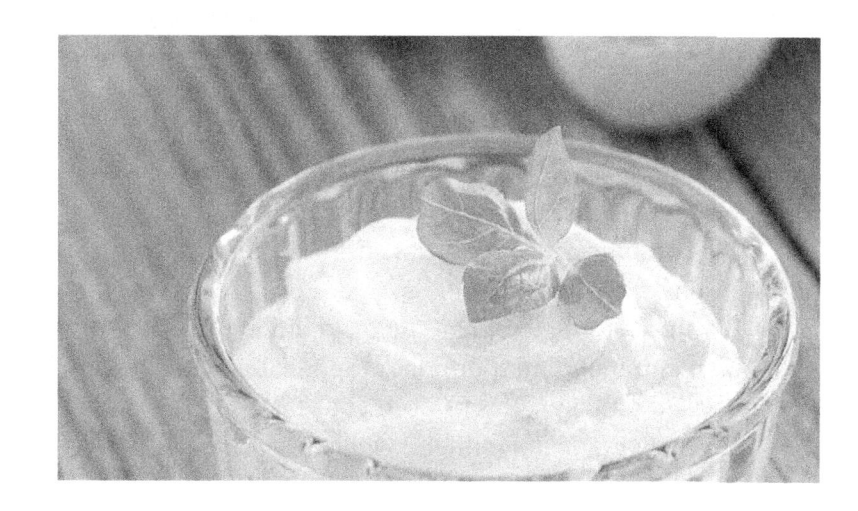

Mayonnaise Cream

(Prep Time: 10 min | Cooking Time: 00 min | Servings 4)

Ingredients:

- 2 egg yolks
- ¾ cup of coconut oil, melted
- ½ cup of olive oil
- 2 teaspoons of fresh lemon juice
- 1 teaspoon of mustard

- Salt

Directions:

1. Combine the egg yolks with lemon juice and mustard in a blender; process and keep blending them smooth while adding the oil gradually.
2. Keep blending them until the mix becomes creamy; add to it a pinch of salt to your taste.
3. Serve your mayonnaise right away or save it in the fridge until ready to use it and enjoy.

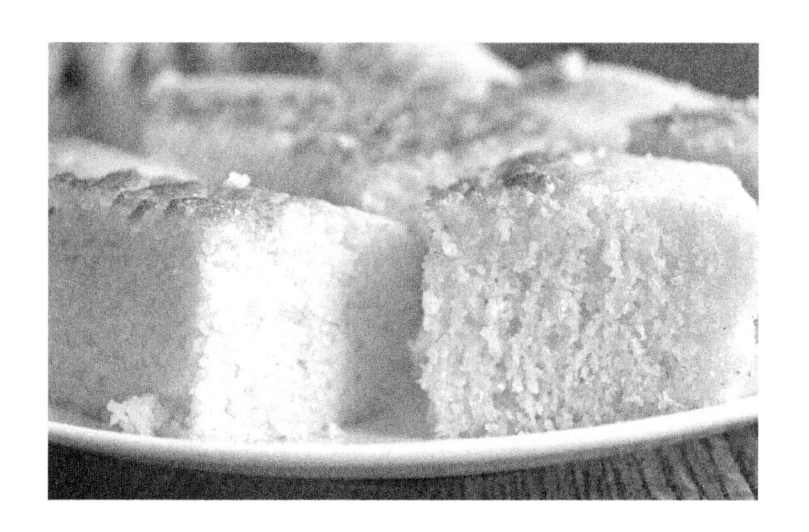

Classic Keto Cornbread

(Prep Time: 10 min | Cooking Time: 26 min | Servings 8)

Ingredients:

- 5 eggs
- 2 cups of almond flour, blanched
- ¼ cup of golden flax meal
- 2 tablespoons of apple cider vinegar
- ½ teaspoon of baking soda

- Salt

Directions:

1. Before you do anything, preheat the oven to 350 F.
2. Combine all the ingredients in a food processor, then pulse them several times until they are well combined.
3. Pour the batter into a lined baking pan and bake it for 24 to 26 min.
4. Once the time is up, allow the cornbread to cool down completely, then serve it and enjoy.

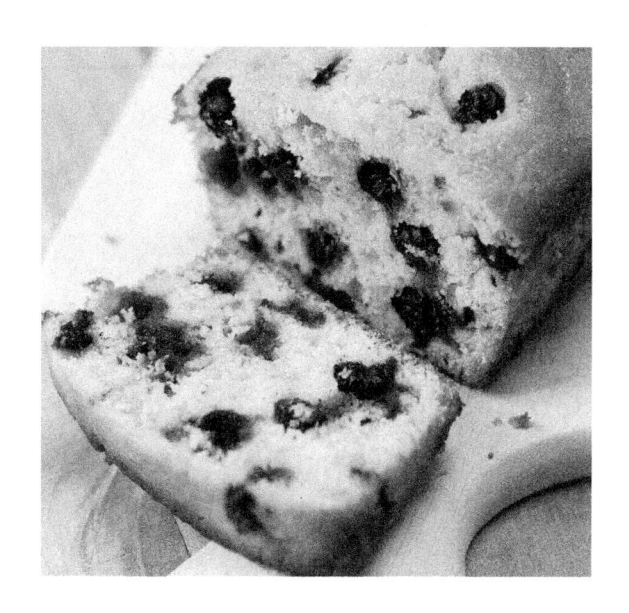

Zesty Blueberry Cake

(Prep Time: 10 min | Cooking Time: 56 min | Servings 8)

Ingredients:

3 cups of almond flour, blanched
6 eggs
1 cup fresh blueberries

- 2 tablespoons of egg white protein powder
- 1 tablespoon of fresh lemon zest, grated
- 1 teaspoon cream of tartar
- ½ teaspoon of baking soda
- ½ teaspoon of vanilla stevia
- Salt

Directions:

1. Before you do anything, preheat the oven to 350 F.
2. Stir the flour with protein powder, lemon zest, cream of tartar, baking soda and a pinch of salt in a large mixing bowl.
3. Transfer the mixture to a food processor, then add to them the eggs with vanilla and stevia; pulse them several times until they become smooth.
4. Pour the batter into a mixing bowl and fold the berries into it.
5. Pour the batter into a greased loaf pan, then bake it for 48 to 56 min.
6. Once the time is up, place the cake aside to cool down, then serve it and enjoy.

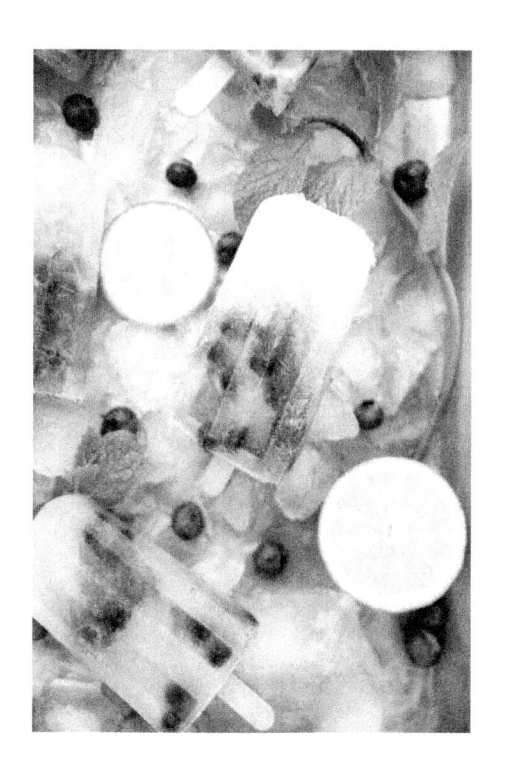

Blue Summer Mojito Pops

(Prep Time: 5 min | Cooking Time: 00 min | Servings 8)

Ingredients:

- 2 cups of water
- ½ cup of blueberries, fresh
- ½ cup of fresh lime juice
- Few mint leaves
- ¼ teaspoon of stevia

Directions:

1. Stir all the ingredients in a large mason jar, then pour into popsicle mold.
2. Freeze the popsicles for 3hr, then serve them and enjoy.

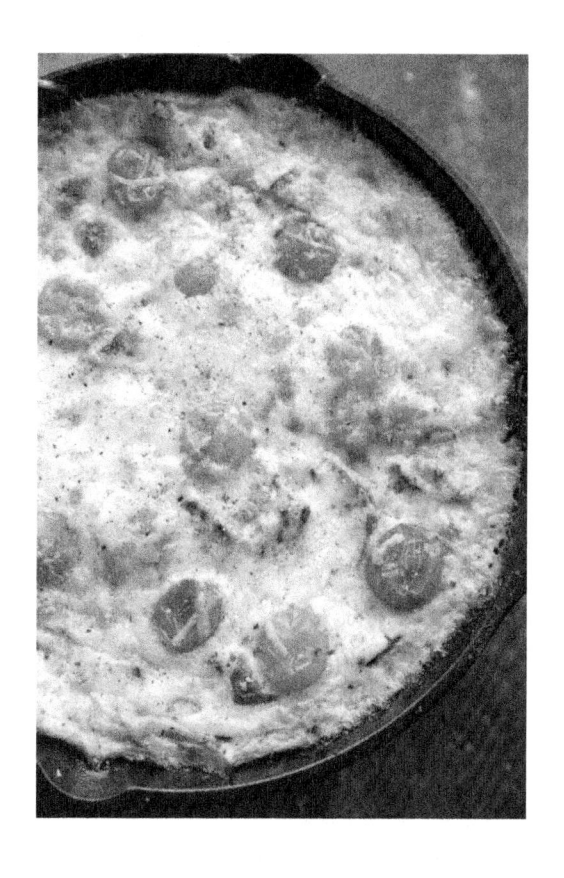

Cheesy Cherries Frittata

(Prep Time: 10 min | Cooking Time: 14 min | Servings 2 to 3)

Ingredients:

- 6 eggs
- 2/3 cup of cherry tomatoes, halved
- 2/3 cup of feta cheese
- ½ yellow onion, finely chopped
- 1 small bunch of spinach, frozen and sliced
- 1 tablespoon of ghee
- Black pepper
- Salt

Directions:

1. Melt the ghee in a large ovenproof skillet, then sauté the onion for 4 min over low medium heat.
2. Whisk the eggs in a large mixing bowl with some salt and pepper.
3. Fold the tomato and spinach into the mix.
4. Pour the egg mix into the hot skillet and sprinkle the cheese on top.
5. Cook the frittata in the oven for 8 to 10 min or until it is done, then serve it warm and enjoy.

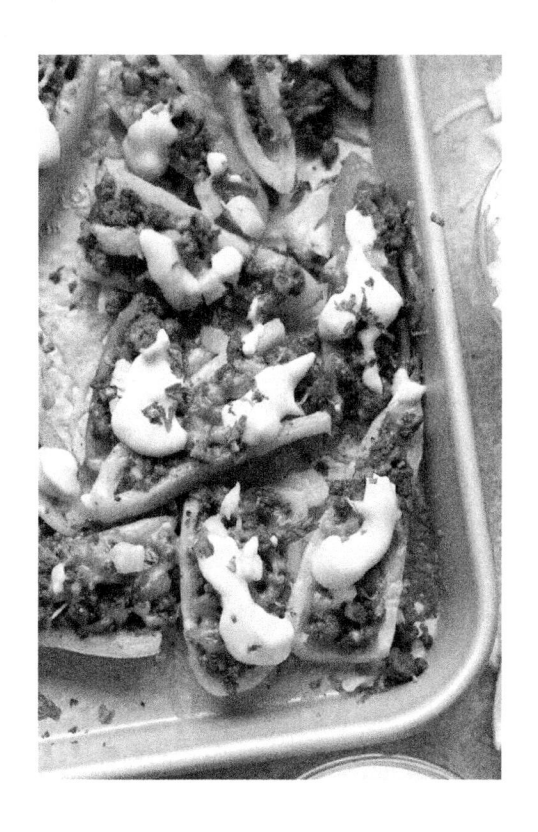

Meaty Pepper Popper Nachos

(Prep Time: 10 min | Cooking Time: 18 min | Servings 4)

Ingredients:

- 1 pound of mini peppers, halved and seeded
- 1 pound of lean beef, minced
- 1 ½ cup of cheddar cheese, shredded
- 1 tablespoon of chili powder
- 1 teaspoon of cumin
- 1 teaspoon of garlic powder
- ½ teaspoon of oregano, dry
- Black pepper
- Salt

Directions:

1. Before you do anything else, preheat the oven to 400 F.
2. Cook the beef in a large pan over medium heat for 8 min.
3. Add the chili powder with garlic, cumin, oregano, some salt and pepper, then cook them for 2 min while stirring all the time.
4. Place the pepper halves on a greased baking sheet, then fill them with the ground beef and top them with the shredded cheese.
5. Bake the pepper nachos in the oven for 8 min until the cheese melts, then serve them warm and enjoy.

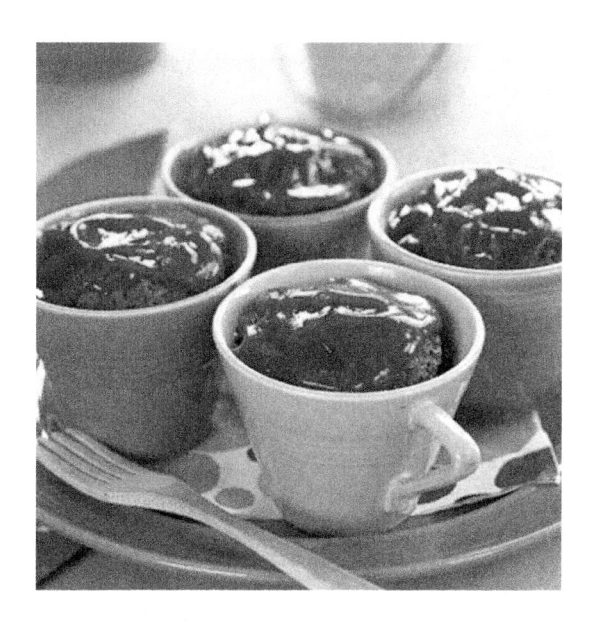

Fall's Meatloaf Cups

(Prep Time: 10 min | Cooking Time: 9 min | Servings 4)

Ingredients:

- 16 ounces of lean beef, minced
- 1 cup of cheddar cheese, shredded

- 12 3 tablespoons of sweet tomato salsa, sugar free
- 1 teaspoon of onion powder
- Black pepper
- Salt

Directions:

1. Combine all the ingredients in a large mixing bowl, then mix them well with your hands.
2. Spoon the mix into 4 greased oven sage mugs then place them in the microwave and cook them for 7 to 9 min.
3. Once the time is up, serve your meatloaf mugs warm with extra salsa and enjoy.

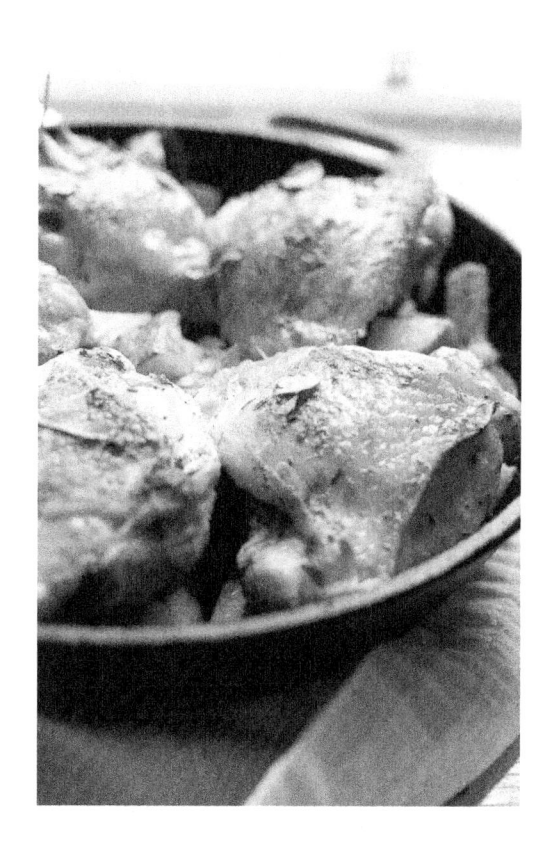

Herbed Crispy Chicken Thighs

(Prep Time: 10 min | Cooking Time: 25 min | Servings 4)

Ingredients:

- 8 chicken thighs, boneless
- 2 tablespoons of ghee
- 2 tablespoons of olive oil
- 2 tablespoons of fresh lemon juice
- 1 tablespoon of fresh thyme, finely chopped
- 2 cloves of garlic, minced
- Black pepper
- Salt

Directions:

1. Mix the chicken thighs with olive oil, lemon juice, thyme, garlic, some salt and pepper.
2. Place the marinated chicken thighs in the fridge to sit for at least 1 h.
3. Once the time is up, drain the chicken thighs from the marinade.
4. Melt the ghee in a large skillet over medium heat, then cook the chicken thighs for 8 to 12 min on each side or until they become golden brown.
5. Drain the chicken thighs, then serve them warm and enjoy.

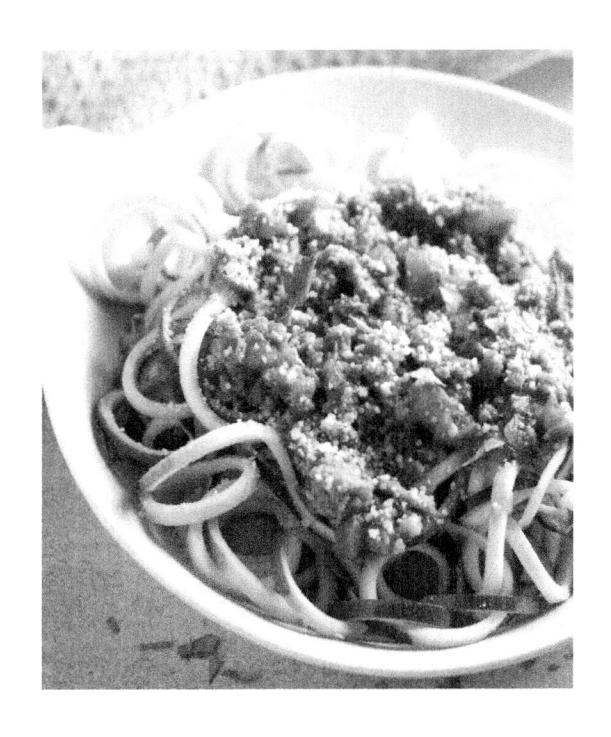

Beef Zoodles Ragu

(Prep Time: 10 min | Cooking Time: 14 min | Servings 4)

Ingredients:

- 2 pounds of lean beef, minced
- 4 zucchinis, spiralized
- ¼ cup of red pesto
- ¼ cup of parsley, finely chopped
- 1 tablespoon of ghee
- Black pepper
- Salt

Directions:

1. Melt the ghee in a large skillet then brown the beef for 7 to 9 min.
2. Add the parsley with pesto, some salt and pepper, then cook them for 5 min while stirring often over medium heat.
3. Once the time is up, serve your Beef Ragu over the Zoodles, then serve it and enjoy.

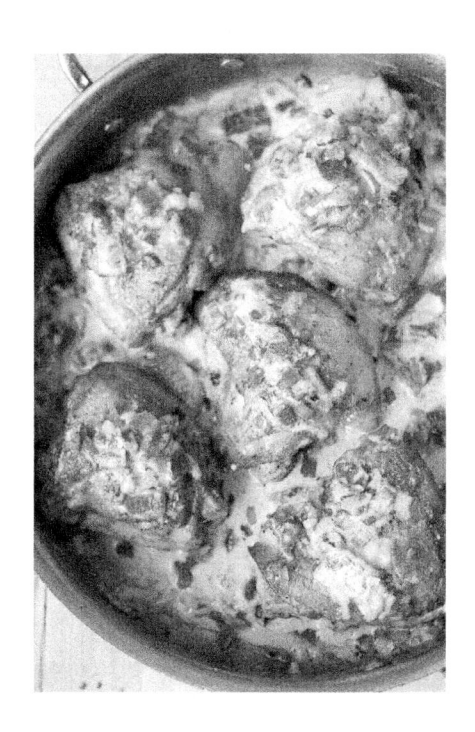

Golden Chicken Thighs with Cream Sauce

(Prep Time: 10 min | Cooking Time: 26 min | Servings 4)

Ingredients:

- 4 chicken thighs, boneless
- 8 ounces of sour cream
- 4 bacon slices, cooked and diced
- 2 tablespoons of butter
- Black pepper
- Salt

Directions:

1. Season the chicken thighs with some salt and pepper.
2. Melt the butter in a large pan, then cook the chicken over medium low heat for 8 to 10 min on each side with the lid on.
3. Once the time is up, turn the heat to medium high and cook them until they become golden brown on each side.
4. Stir the cream into the skillet then turn off the heat and sprinkle the bacon pieces on top.
5. Allow the chicken skillet to sit for 4 min, then serve it warm and enjoy.

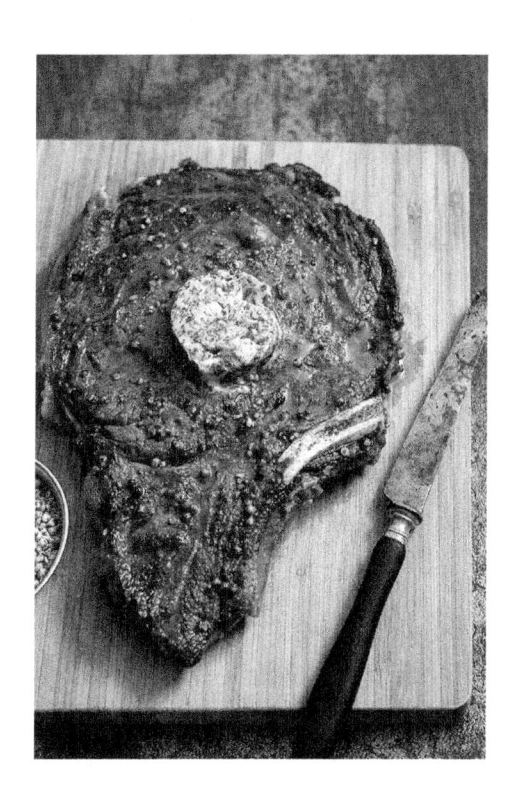

Seared Steak with Keto Butter Sauce

(Prep Time: 12 min | Cooking Time: 24 min | Servings 2)

Ingredients:

- 14 to 15 oz (2) rib eye steaks
- 4 tablespoons of parsley, finely chopped
- 4 tablespoons of ghee
- 1 teaspoon of coriander seeds
- 2 cloves of garlic, minced
- 1 teaspoon of olive oil
- 1 teaspoon of lemon juice
- 2 teaspoons of lemon zest, grated
- Black pepper
- Salt

Directions:

1. Stir the coriander seeds with lemon juice and olive oil in a small bowl, then massage it into the steaks.
2. Season the steaks with some salt and pepper.
3. Melt 1 tablespoon ghee in a heavy pan, then cook the steaks over medium heat for 4 min on each side until they become golden brown.
4. Lower the heat and keep cooking the steaks for 6 to 7 min on each side over low heat or until the steak is done to your liking.
5. Once the time is up, mix the parsley with 3 tablespoons of ghee, garlic, lemon zest and a pinch of salt in a small mixing bowl to make the sauce.
6. Allow the steaks to rest for 5 min, then serve them with the sauce on the side and enjoy.

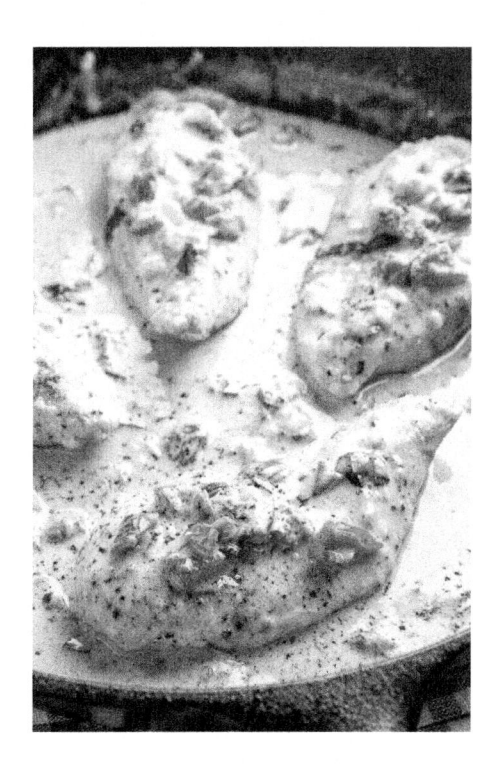

Sunny Chicken Cream Skillet

(Prep Time: 10 min | Cooking Time: 20 min | Servings 4 to 6)

Ingredients:

- 1 ½ pounds of chicken breasts, halved
- 1 cup of heavy cream
- 1 cup of spinach, finely chopped
- ½ cup of chicken broth
- ½ cup of sundried tomato, chopped
- ½ cup of parmesan cheese, shredded
- 2 tablespoons of olive oil
- 1 teaspoon of Italian seasoning
- 1 teaspoon of garlic powder
- Black pepper
- Salt

Directions:

1. Season the chicken breasts with some salt and pepper.
2. Heat the oil in a large pan, then brown in it the chicken breasts for 4 to 6 min on each side until they are done.
3. Drain the chicken breasts and place them aside.
4. Add the cream with cheese, broth, Italian seasoning, garlic powder, a pinch of salt and pepper to the same skillet, then whisk them over medium low heat until the cheese melts.
5. Add the sundried tomato with spinach to the pan and cook them for 1 min.

6. Place the chicken breasts back in the skillet and spoon the sauce over them; then cook them for an extra 2 min.

7. Serve your sunny chicken skillet warm and enjoy.

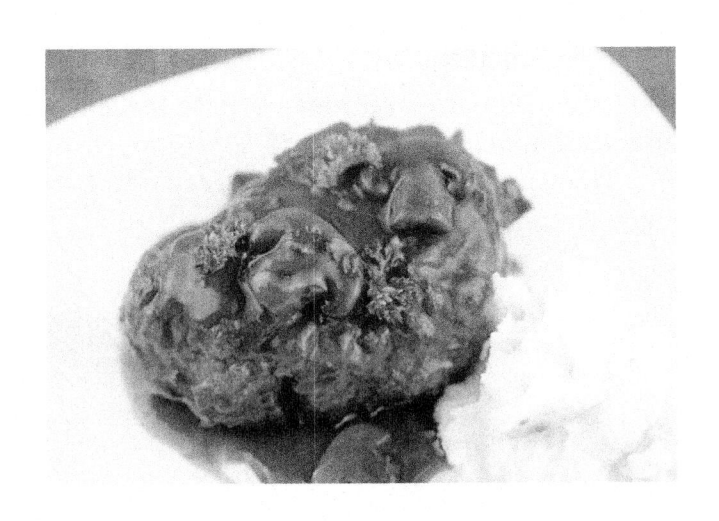

Salisbury Steak Patties with Mushroom Gravy

(Prep Time: 15 min | Cooking Time: 20 min | Servings 6)

Ingredients:

- Pound of lean beef chuck, minced
- 2 cups of button mushrooms, sliced
- 1 cup of yellow onion, thinly sliced
- ¾ cup of almond flour

- ¾ cup of beef broth
- ¼ cup of sour cream
- 4 tablespoons of butter
- 1 tablespoon of parsley, finely chopped
- 1 tablespoon and teaspoon of Worcestershire sauce
- ½ teaspoon of garlic powder
- Black pepper
- Salt

Directions:

1. Before you do anything preheat the oven to 375 F.
2. Combine the beef chuck with almond flour, ¼ cup of broth, parsley, 1 tablespoon of Worcestershire sauce, garlic powder, some salt and pepper in a large mixing bowl.
3. Knead the ingredients with your hands to combine the flavors.
4. Shape the mix into 6 thick patties and place them on a lined-up baking sheet, then bake them for 19 min.
5. Melt the butter in a large skillet, then sauté in it the mushroom for 2 to 3 min on each side.
6. Stir the onion into the skillet with a pinch of salt and pepper them cook them for 6 min.
7. Add 1 teaspoon of Worcestershire sauce with ½ cup of broth, then cook them for an extra 3 min.

8. Stir the sour cream into the sauce and turn off the heat.

9. Serve your baked steak patties warm with the mushroom gravy and enjoy.

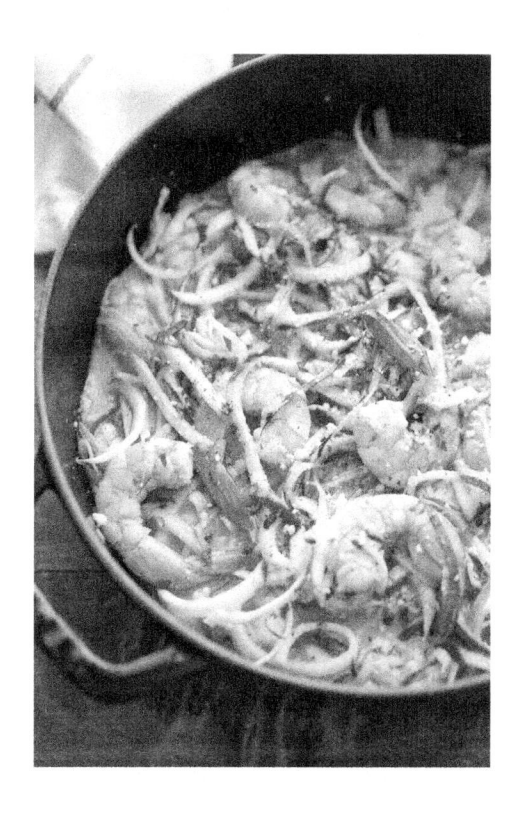

Shrimp Zoodles Sauté

(Prep Time: 15 min | Cooking Time: 20 min | Servings 4)

Ingredients:

- ¾ pound of shrimp, peeled and deveined
- 2 zucchinis, spiralized
- The juice of 1 lemon
- The zest of 1 lemon, grated
- 1 tablespoons of olive oil
- 2 cloves of garlic, minced
- Black pepper
- Salt

Directions:

1. Heat the olive oil with garlic, lemon juice and zest in a large skillet.
2. Add the shrimp with a pinch of salt and pepper then cook it for 1 min on each side.
3. Stir the zucchini into the skillet and cook for 2 to 4 min while stirring all the time.
4. Serve your shrimp and zucchini skillet warm and enjoy.

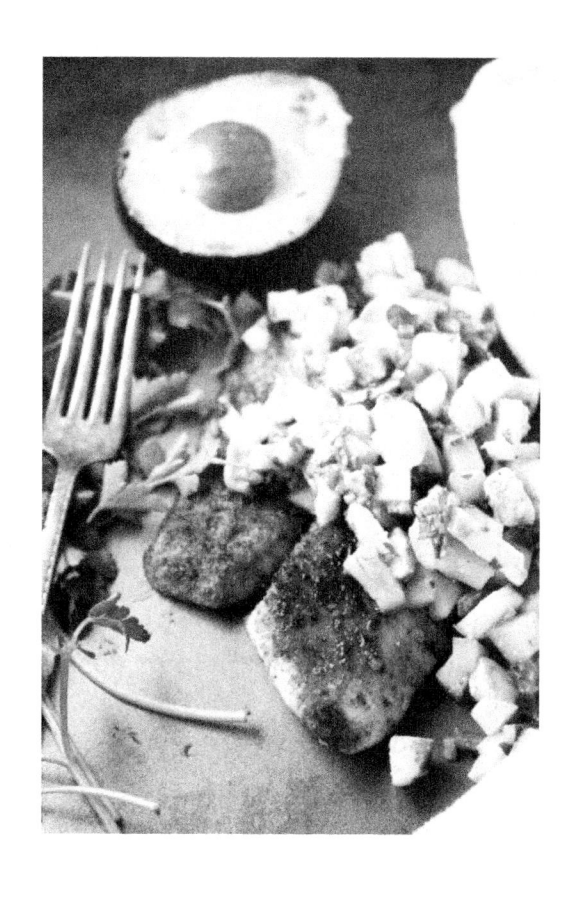

Seared Cajun Salmon

(Prep Time: 10 min | Cooking Time: 14 min | Servings 4)

Ingredients:

- 4 (6 oz) salmon fillets
- 1 tablespoon of olive oil
- 4 teaspoon of Cajun seasoning
- Black pepper
- Salt

Directions:

1. Season the salmon fillets with some salt and pepper, then rub the Cajun seasoning into them.
2. Heat the oil in a large skillet, then cook in it the fillets 4 to 7 min on each side or until it is done to your liking.
3. Serve your salmon fillets warm and enjoy.

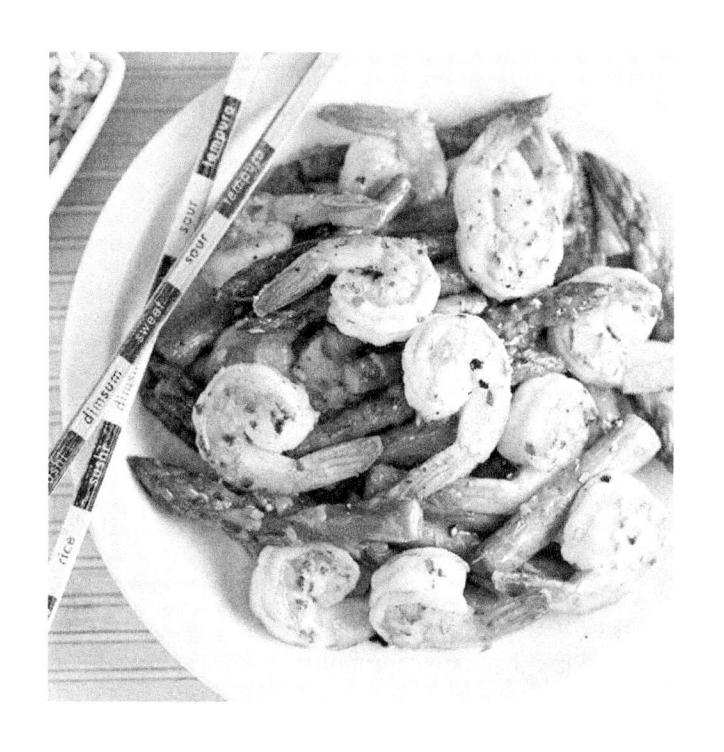

Roasted Shrimp and Asparagus

(Prep Time: 5 min | Cooking Time: 12 min | Servings 4)

Ingredients:

- 1 ½ pound of shrimp, peeled and deveined
- 1 pound of asparagus, trimmed and halved
- 3 tablespoons of butter
- 3 cloves of garlic, minced
- 2 tablespoons of olive oil
- 1 ½ tablespoon of fresh lemon juice
- ¼ teaspoon of paprika
- Black pepper
- Salt

Directions:

1. Toss all the ingredients in a mixing bowl except for the butter.
2. Pick the asparagus pieces, then spread it on the side of a lined up and greased baking sheet.
3. Cook the asparagus in the oven for 5 min.
4. Once the time is up, place the shrimp on the other side of the pan.
5. Slice the butter into small cubes, then spread them over the asparagus and shrimp.
6. Roast them in the oven for 7 min, then serve them warm and enjoy.

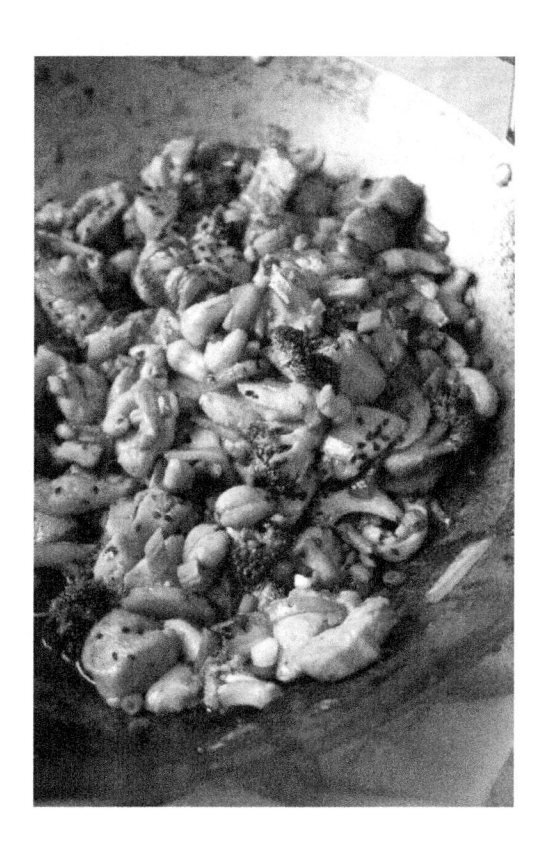

Nutty Chicken and Broccoli Stir Fry

(Prep Time: 10 min | Cooking Time: 10 min | Servings 4)

Ingredients:

- 4 chicken thighs, cut into bite size pieces
- ½ cup of broccoli florets, chopped
- ¼ cup of cashews, toasted
- ¼ cup of onion, finely chopped
- 2 tablespoons of canola oil
- 1 ½ tablespoon of soy sauce
- 1 tablespoon of rice wine vinegar
- 1 tablespoon of garlic, minced
- ½ tablespoon of chili garlic sauce
- Black pepper
- Salt

Directions:

1. Place a large skillet over medium heat, then heat the oil in it.
2. Add the chicken to the skillet and cook it for 6 min.
3. Stir the remaining ingredients into the skillet with some salt and pepper, then cook them for 3 to 4 min while stirring often.
4. Serve your stir fry warm and enjoy.

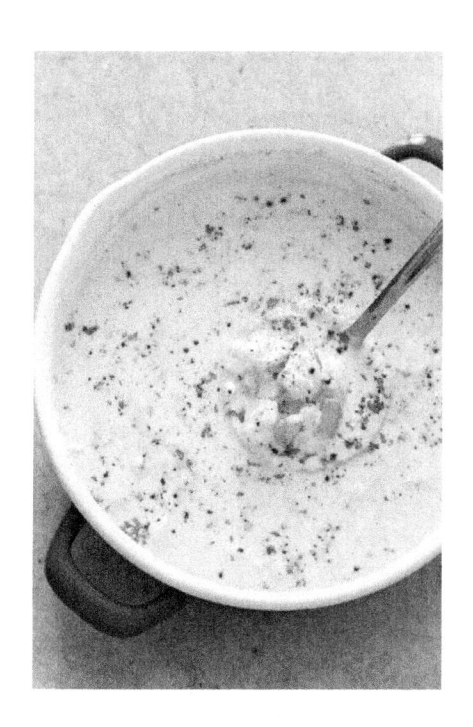

Creamy Cauliflower Chowder

(Prep Time: 10 min | Cooking Time: 30 min | Servings 4)

Ingredients:

- 1 medium head of cauliflower, cut into florets

- 2 ½ cup of veggies broth
- ½ cup of yellow onion, diced
- ½ cup of carrot, diced
- ¼ cup of cream cheese
- 3 cloves of garlic, minced
- 1 tablespoon of butter
- ½ teaspoon of dry oregano
- Black pepper
- Salt

Directions:

1. Melt the butter in a soup pot, then sauté the onion with garlic for 4 min.
2. Stir the carrot with 1 ½ cups broth, cauliflower, some salt and pepper, then cook them until they start boiling.
3. Lower the heat and simmer the soup for 16 min.
4. Turn off the heat and allow the soup to cool down for a while, then transfer 1/3 of it to a food processor and blend it smooth.
5. Pour the blended soup back to the pot, then stir into it the remaining broth with cream cheese.
6. Simmer the soup for 8 to 10 min over low medium heat, then serve it warm and enjoy.

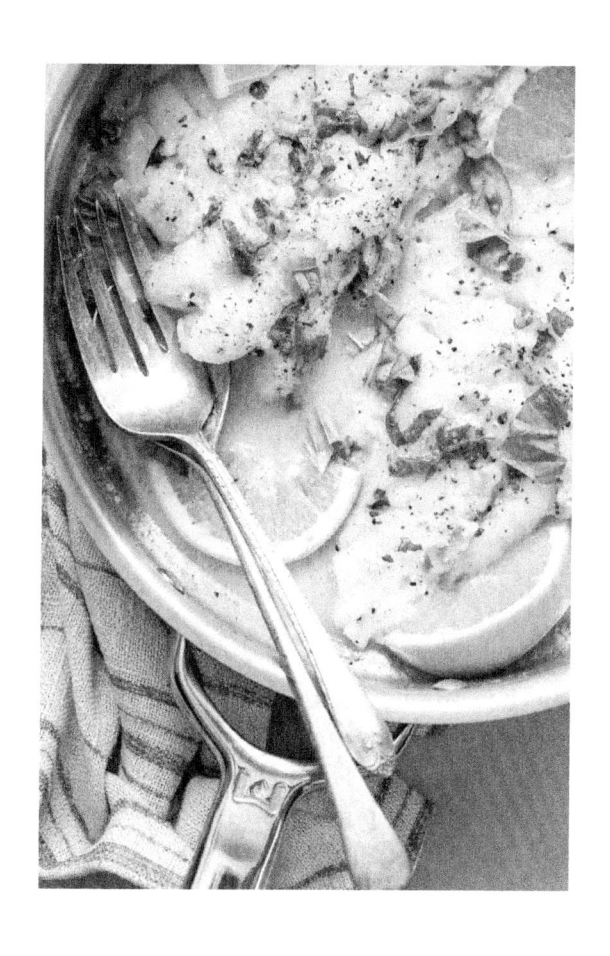

Seasoned Cod Skillet

(Prep Time: 5 min | Cooking Time: 7 min | Servings 2 to 4)

Ingredients:

- 1 ½ pound of cod fillets
- 6 tablespoons of butter
- ½ teaspoon of lemon zest, grated
- ¼ teaspoon of paprika
- ¼ teaspoon of garlic powder
- Black pepper
- Salt

Directions:

1. Season the cod fillets with some salt and pepper.
2. Mix the paprika with lemon zest and garlic powder in a small bowl, then season the cod fillets with it.
3. Melt half of the butter in a large skillet, then cook in it the cod fillets for 2 min.
4. Flip the cod fillets and add the remaining butter, then cook them for 3 to 5 min over medium heat.
5. Once the time is up, serve your cod fillets skillet warm with your favorite toppings and enjoy.

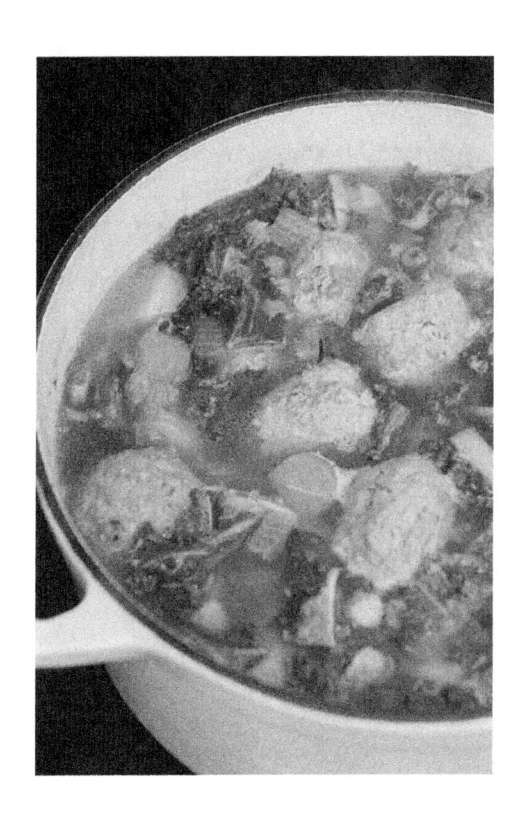

Meatballs Wedding Soup

(Prep Time: 15 min | Cooking Time: 30 min | Servings 4)

Ingredients:

- 1 pound of lean turkey, minced
- 6 cups of chicken broth
- 1 small yellow onion, diced
- 4 carrots, diced
- 1 bunch of kale, torn
- 1 egg, beaten
- 3 tablespoons of cassava flour
- 4 tablespoons of ghee
- 2 tablespoons of mixed herbs, finely chopped
- 3 cloves of garlic, minced
- 2 bay leaves
- Black pepper
- Salt

Directions:

1. Combine the lean turkey with cassava flour, herbs, 2 minced cloves of garlic, egg, some salt and pepper, then mix them well.
2. Shape the mix into bite size meatballs.
3. Melt 2 tablespoons of ghee in a large pan, then cook in it the meatballs in batches for 3 to 5 min until they become golden brown.
4. Melt the remaining ghee in a soup pot, then sauté the onion with 1 clove of garlic and carrot for 6 min.

5. Add the cooked meatballs with broth, bay leaves, some salt and pepper, then cook them until they start boiling.

6. Lower the heat and simmer the soup for 6 min.

7. Stir the kale into the soup, then cook it for 8 min.

8. Once the time is up, adjust the seasoning of the soup, then serve it warm and enjoy.

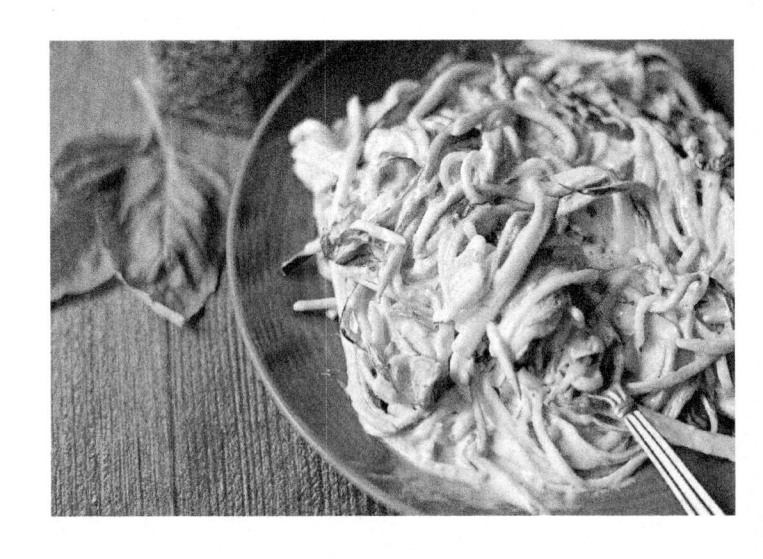

Creamy Keto Alfredo

(Prep Time: 5 min | Cooking Time: 6 min | Servings 3 to 4)

Ingredients:

- 4 zucchinis, spiralized
- 4 ounces of cream cheese
- ¼ cup of parmesan cheese, grated
- 2 tablespoons of milk

- 2 tablespoons of oily sundried tomato, drained and chopped
- 1 tablespoon of butter
- 1 clove of garlic, minced
- Black pepper
- Salt

Directions:

1. Melt the butter in a large skillet over medium heat, then sauté in it the garlic until it becomes golden.
2. Stir the milk with cream cheese until they melt.
3. Stir the zucchini with sundried tomato to the skillet and stir it to coat with the sauce.
4. Add the parmesan cheese and stir them until the cheese melts.
5. Serve your creamy Alfred warm and enjoy.

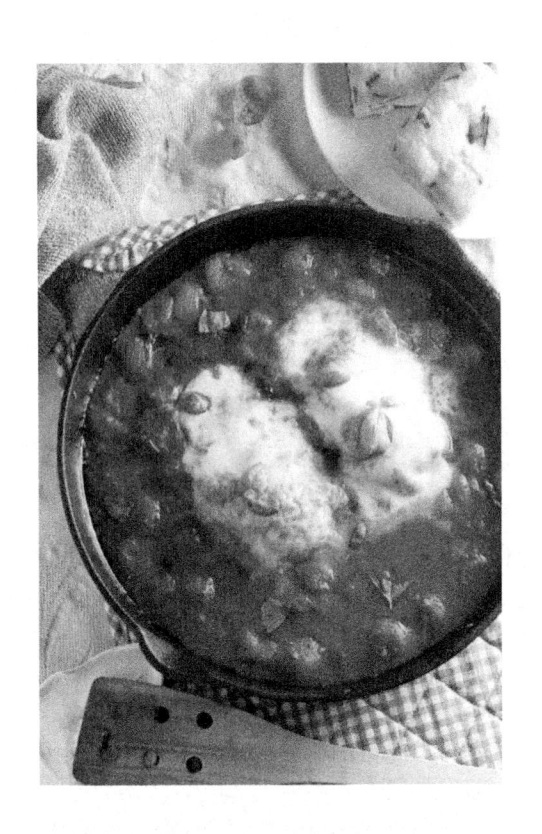

Cheesy and Saucy Chicken Breasts

(Prep Time: 10 min | Cooking Time: 30 min | Servings 4)

Ingredients:

- 4 small chicken breasts
- 4 mozzarella slices
- 14 ounces of canned tomato, crushed
- ½ cup of yellow onion, finely chopped
- ¼ cup of water
- 1 tablespoon of garlic, minced
- 1 tablespoon of olive oil
- 1 tablespoon of pesto
- ½ teaspoon of Italian seasoning
- Black pepper
- Salt

Directions:

1. Heat the oil in a large skillet over medium heat.
2. Cook the chicken for 4 to 6 min on each side until it is no longer pink.
3. Drain the chicken breasts and place them aside.
4. Before you do anything else preheat the oven broiler.
5. Stir the garlic with onion in the same skillet where the chicken was and cook them for 3 min.
6. Cook them for 3 min until they soften, then add to them the crushed tomato with spices.

7. Bring them to a boil, then put on the lid and cook them for 11 min over low heat.

8. Place the chicken breasts in the sauce, then place a slice of cheese on top of each one.

9. Place the chicken skillet in the oven and broil it for 2 to 3 min.

10. Once the time is up, serve your chicken skillet warm and enjoy.

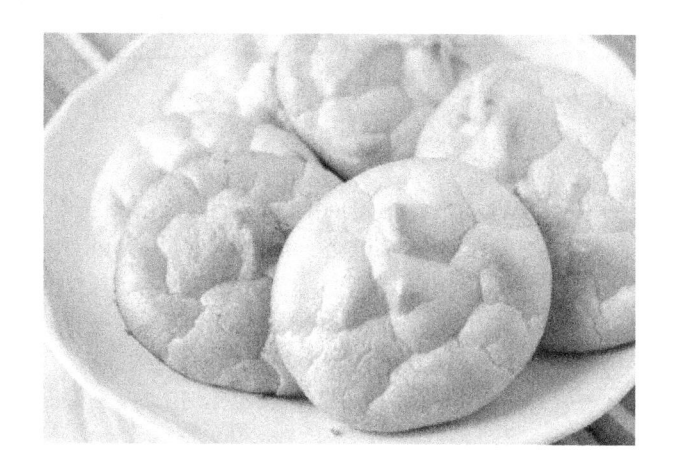

Rosemary Cloud Flat Buns

(Prep Time: 10 min | Cooking Time: 36 min | Servings 6)

Ingredients:

- 3 eggs
- 3 tablespoons of Greek yogurt
- ½ teaspoon of dry rosemary
- ½ teaspoon of garlic powder
- ¼ teaspoon cream of tartar
- Salt

Directions:

1. Before you do anything preheat the oven to 300 F.
2. Place the egg whites in a large mixing bowl, then beat them with cream of tartar until their stiff peaks.
3. Whisk the egg yolks with rosemary, yogurt, garlic powder and a pinch of salt.
4. Add the egg white gradually and fold it gently into the egg yolk mix.
5. Spoon the mix into a lined-up baking sheet in the shape of 6 mounds.
6. Bake the cloud buns in the oven for 36 min.
7. Once the time is up, turn off the heat and open the oven door, then let it cool down for 45 min.
8. Pull out the buns from the oven and place them aside to cool down completely, then serve them and enjoy.

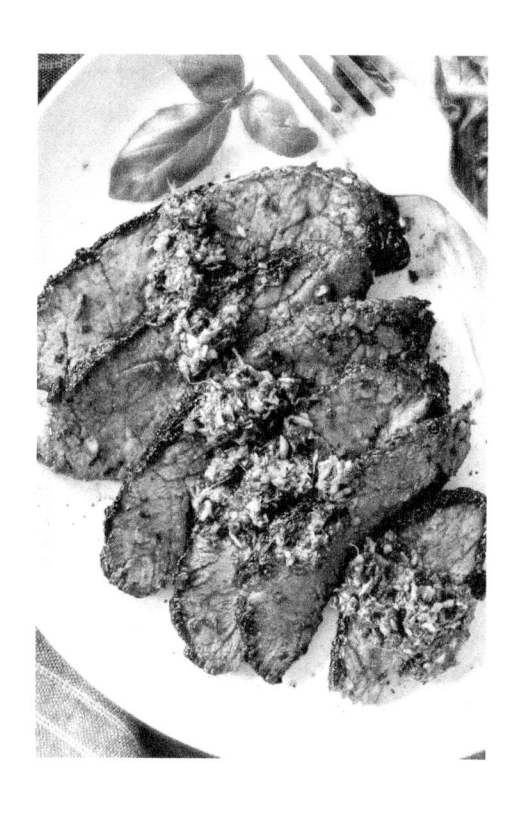

Herbed Tri-Tip

(Prep Time: 10 min | Cooking Time: 38 min | Servings 4 to 6)

Ingredients:

- 2 pounds tri-tip steak
- 2 cups of parsley, finely chopped
- ½ cup and 2 tbsp of olive oil
- ½ cup of cilantro, finely chopped
- ¼ cup of red wine vinegar
- 1 tablespoon of paprika
- 1 tablespoon of agave nectar
- 2 cloves of garlic, minced
- Black pepper
- Salt

Directions:

1. Mix the paprika with 2 tablespoons of olive and tablespoons of parsley in a small mixing bowl.
2. Season the steak with some salt and pepper.
3. Rub the paprika mix all over the steak, then place it in the fridge for 1 h or more.
4. Before you do anything preheat the grill.
5. Put the steak on indirect heat and cover it with the grill lid, then let it cook for 32 min.
6. Once the time is up, transfer the steak to the direct heat, then cook it for 2 to 4 min on each side.
7. Mix the remaining parsley in a mixing bowl with ½ cup of olive oil, cilantro, vinegar, agave nectar and garlic, then mix them well to make the sauce.
8. Serve the herbs sauce over the steak and enjoy.

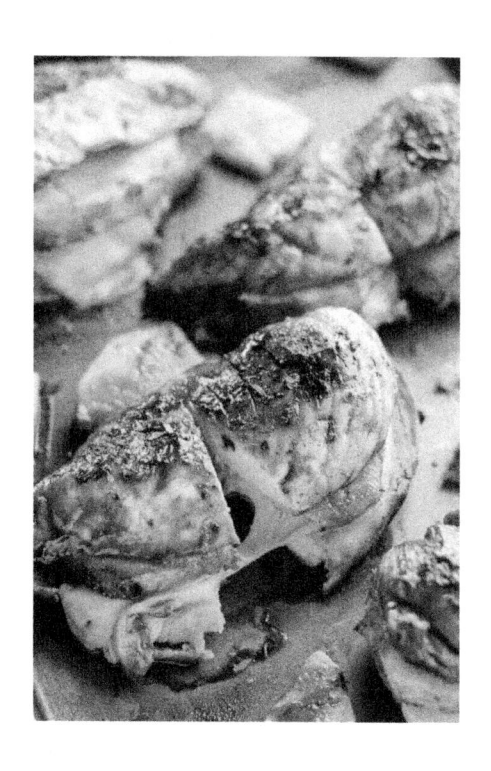

Black Forest Stuffed Chicken Breasts

(Prep Time: 10 min | Cooking Time: 16 min | Servings 4)

Ingredients:

- 4 chicken breasts
- 4 slices of gruyere cheese
- 4 slices of black forest ham
- 1 tablespoon of olive oil
- Black pepper
- Salt

Directions:

1. Before you do anything preheat the oven to 400 F.
2. Cut a slit on the side of each chicken breast creating a pocket in it, then stuff each one of them with 1 slice of cheese and 1 slice of ham.
3. Season the chicken breasts with some salt and pepper.
4. Coat the stuffed chicken breasts with olive oil, then place them on a baking sheet and cook them in the oven for 14 to 16 min.
5. Once the time is up, serve your chicken breasts warm and enjoy.

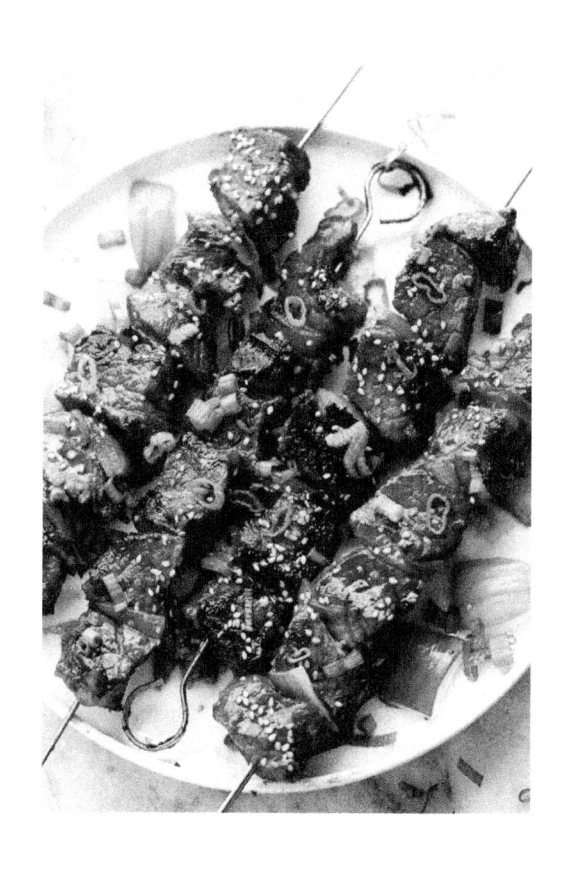

Glazed Teriyaki Skewers

(Prep Time: 10 min | Cooking Time: 8 min | Servings 2)

Ingredients:

- 14 ounces of lean steak, diced
- 1 red onion, diced
- 1 tablespoon of soy sauce
- 1 tablespoon of mirin
- 1 tablespoon of sherry vinegar
- 1 teaspoon of stevia
- 1 teaspoon of soy sauce
- 1 teaspoon of olive oil
- Black pepper
- Salt

Directions:

1. Stir the mirin with vinegar, soy sauce, olive oil, and stevia in a small bowl to make the marinade.
2. Pour the marinade all over the steak and stir them to coat, then place them in the fridge to marinate for 1 h or more.
3. Grease a frying pan with some oil or ghee and heat it over medium heat.
4. Thread the steak onto wooden skewers while alternating between them and the onion, then cook them in the hot pan for 2 to 4 min on each side.
5. Once the time is up, serve your skewers warm and enjoy.

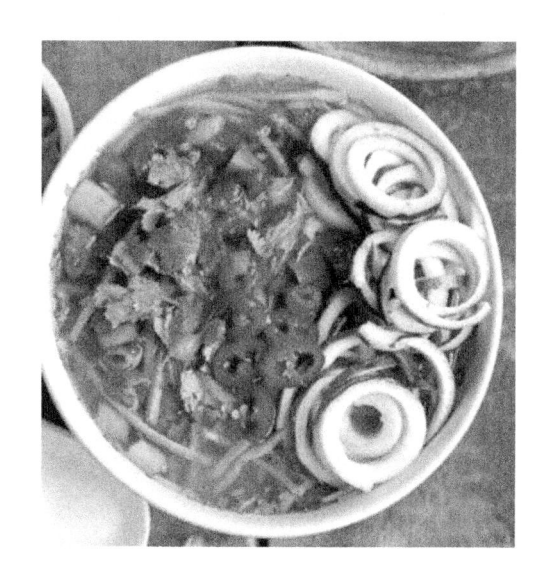

Spiralized Bacon Soup

(Prep Time: 10 min | Cooking Time: 25 min | Servings 4 to 6)

Ingredients:

- 6 cups of chicken broth
- 1 parsnip, spiralized
- 1 turnip, peeled and spiralized
- 1 large carrot, spiralized

- 5 ounces of smoked bacon, diced
- 5 tablespoons of olive oil
- 1 stalk of celery, diced
- 2 cloves of garlic, minced
- 2 sprigs of oregano
- 2 sprigs of fresh thyme
- 1 bay leaf
- Black pepper
- Salt

Directions:

1. Heat 1 tablespoon of over medium heat in a soup pot, then sauté in it the bacon for 6 min.
2. Add the onion with the remaining oil and cook them for 7 min, then stir in the garlic and cook them for another minute.
3. Add the oregano with thyme, bay leaf and broth, then simmer the soup for 16 min.
4. Stir the spiralized veggies into the soup and season them with some salt and pepper.
5. Turn off the heat and allow the soup for sit for 6 min, then serve it warm and enjoy.

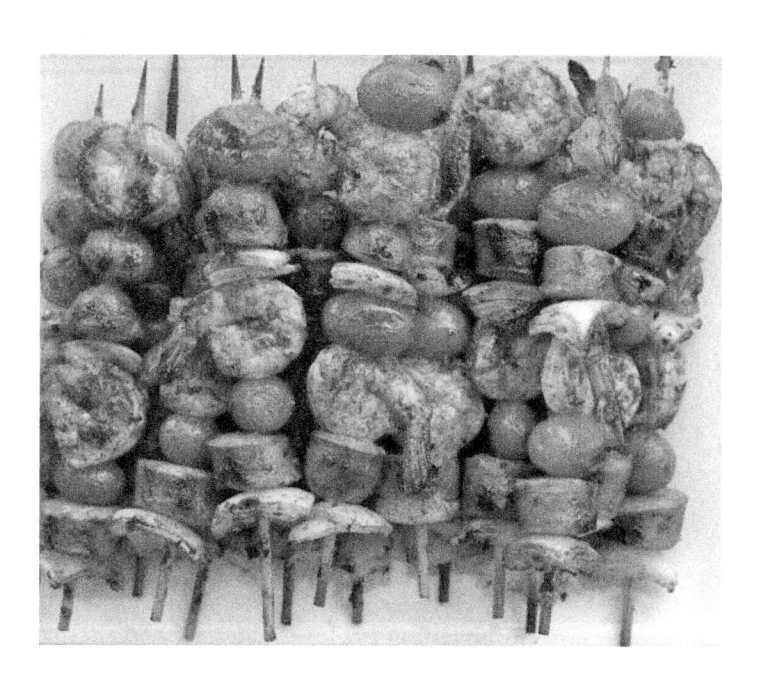

Glazed Shrimp Skewers

(Prep Time: 15 min | Cooking Time: 20 min | Servings 4)

Ingredients:

12 inches long andouille sausages, smoked and sliced

- 12 large shrimp, peeled and deveined
- ¾ cup of olive oil
- 12 cherry tomatoes
- 12 onion wedges
- 2 tablespoons of fresh thyme, finely chopped
- 3 cloves of garlic, minced
- 5 teaspoons of paprika
- 4 teaspoons of sherry wine vinegar
- Black pepper
- Salt

Directions:

1. Before you do anything preheat the grill and grease it.
2. Mix the garlic with thyme, olive oil, paprika, vinegar, some salt and pepper in a small mixing bowl to make the marinade.
3. Thread the sausage pieces with shrimp, cherry tomato and onion wedges into skewers while alternating between them.
4. Use a brush to brush the skewers with the marinade.
5. Grill the skewers while basting them every once in a while for 3 to 4 min on each side, then serve them warm and enjoy.

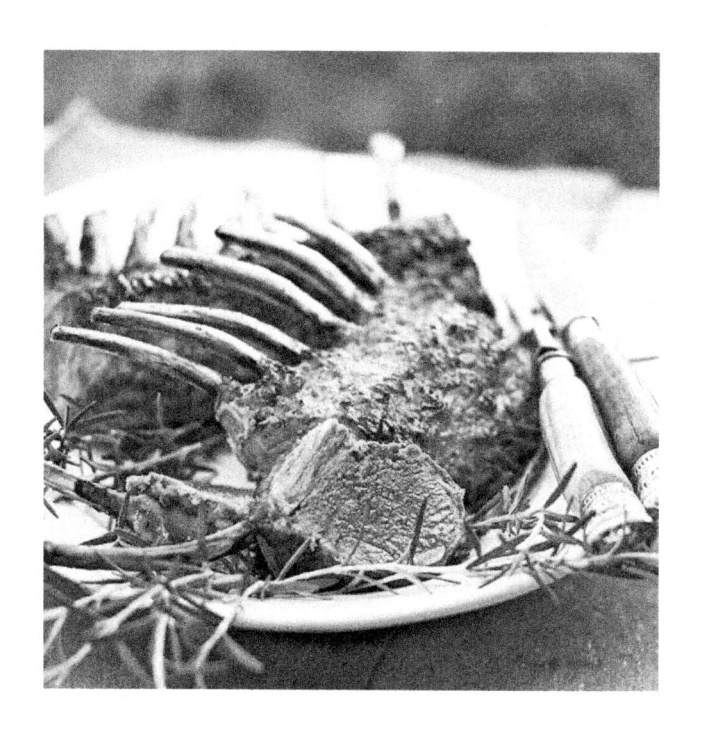

Grilled Rosy Chops

(Prep Time: 15 min | Cooking Time: 20 min | Servings 4)

Ingredients:

- 8 lamb chops
- 1 tablespoon of fresh rosemary, finely chopped
- 2 tablespoons of olive oil
- 2 cloves of garlic, minced
- Black pepper
- Salt

Directions:

1. Mix the rosemary with olive oil and garlic in a small bowl.
2. Season the lamb chops with some salt and pepper, then rub them with the rosemary mix.
3. Place the lamb chops aside to sit for 30 min to 1 h.
4. Preheat the grill and grease it, then grill the chops for 4 to 6 min on each side
5. Serve them warm and enjoy.

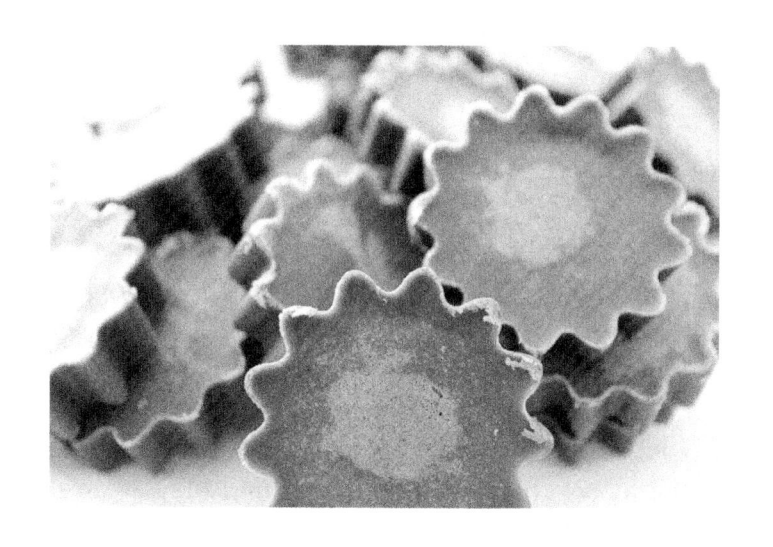

Macadamia and Chocolate Bombs

(Prep Time: 15 min | Cooking Time: 20 min | Servings 4)

Ingredients:

- 4 ounces of macadamia, finely chopped
- ¼ cup of heavy cream
- 2 ounces of cocoa butter
- 2 tablespoons of cocoa powder

- 2 tablespoons of swerve sweetener
- Salt

Directions:

1. Stir the cocoa butter in a saucepan over steamer until it melts, then add the cocoa powder and whisk them well.
2. Add the swerve sweetener, then stir them again until they melt.
3. Fold the macadamia nuts into the batter, then add the heavy cream and stir them until they are well combined.
4. Pour the mix into silicon molds, then freeze them until they become hard
5. Serve them and enjoy.

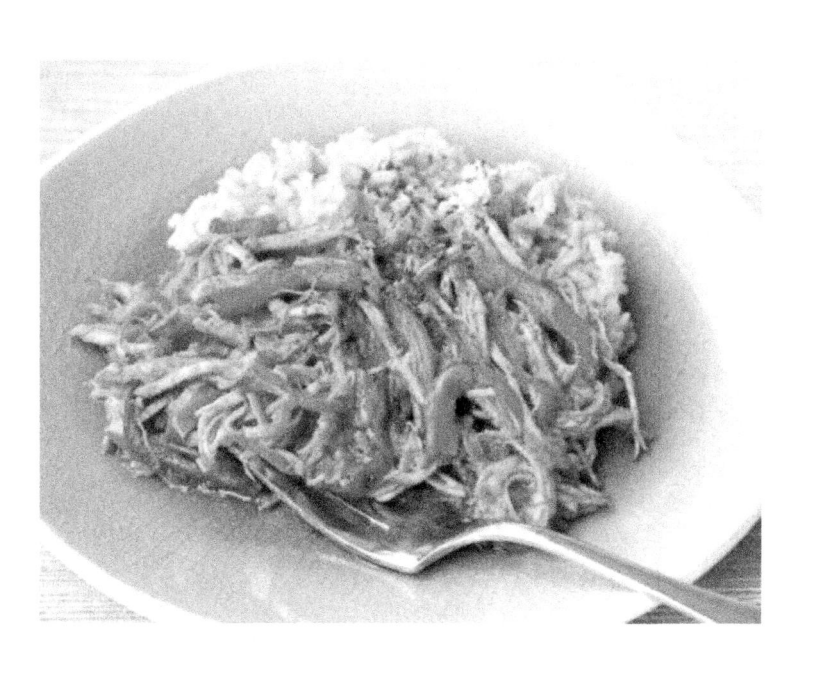

Juicy Ropa Vieja

(Prep Time: 15 min | Cooking Time: 20 min | Servings 6)

Ingredients:

3 pounds of chicken breasts, cut into pieces
12 ounces of tomato paste

- 3 bell peppers, thinly sliced
- ¼ cup of olive oil
- ¼ cup of parsley, finely chopped
- 2 tablespoons of coconut oil
- 1 tablespoon of white wine vinegar
- 1 tablespoon of fresh oregano, finely chopped
- 1 tablespoon of garlic powder
- 1 tablespoon of cumin
- 3 cloves of garlic, minced
- Black pepper
- Salt

Directions:

1. Stir all the ingredients in a slow cooker, then put on the lid and cook them for 6 h.
2. Once the time is up, drain the chicken pieces and shred them, then stir them back into the pot.
3. Serve your ropa vieja warm and enjoy.

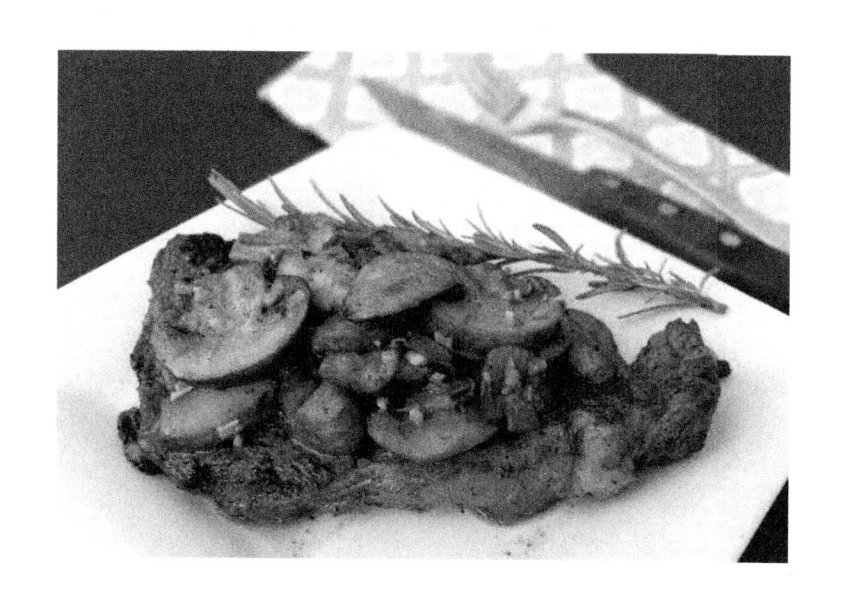

Seared Steak with Mushroom

(Prep Time: 10 min | Cooking Time: 14 min | Servings 4)

Ingredients:

- 4 New York Strip Steaks
- 5 cups of wild mushrooms, sliced
- 2 tablespoons of butter
- 1 tablespoon of olive oil

- 2 cloves of garlic, minced
- Black pepper
- Salt

Directions:

1. Heat the olive oil in a large pan.
2. Season the steaks with some salt and pepper, then sear them in the hot oil for 4 to 6 min on each side, then drain them and place them aside.
3. Melt the butter in the same pan and sauté in it the garlic for 1 min.
4. Stir in the sliced mushroom and cook them for 3 to 6 min while stirring often.
5. Adjust the seasoning of the mushrooms, then serve with the steaks and enjoy.

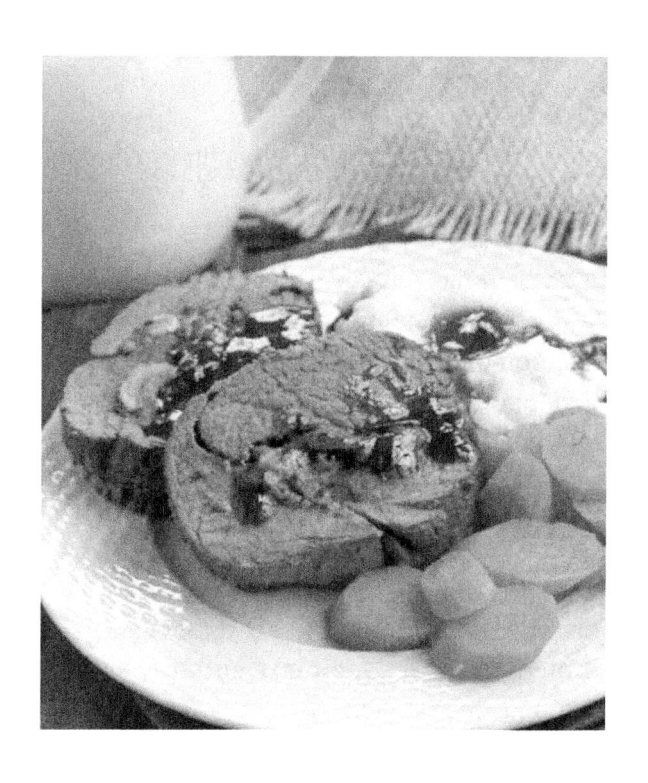

Fancy Stuffed Beef Heart

(Prep Time: 15 min | Cooking Time: 36 min | Servings 6)

Ingredients:

- 1 large beef heart
- 6 bacon slices, thick
- 1 ¼ pound of button mushrooms, finely chopped
- ¼ pound of spinach
- 1 yellow onion, finely chopped
- 3 cloves of garlic, minced
- ½ teaspoon of cinnamon
- ¼ teaspoon of nutmeg powder
- Black pepper
- Salt

Directions:

1. Before you do anything preheat the oven to 275 F.
2. Slice the beef heart open in a butterfly style, then rinse it and clean it well.
3. Pat the beef heart dry and place it aside.
4. Cook the bacon in a large pan over medium heat until it becomes crisp, then drain it and place it aside.
5. Add the mushroom with onion and a pinch of salt to the same skillet with the remaining bacon grease, then sauté them for 6 min.
6. Chop the bacon and add it to the pan with the garlic, cinnamon, nutmeg powder and a pinch of pepper, then cook them for another minute.
7. Add the spinach and cook for another minute.
8. Place the beef heart on a lined baking sheet with the open side facing up, then spoon the mushroom to it and spread it over it.

9. Roll the beef heart over the filling, then wrap kitchen twine around to tie it and prevent the filling from coming out.
10. Melt some fat or bacon grease in a large pan, then sear in it the heart beef for 3 to 5 min on each side until it becomes golden brown.
11. Drain the beef heart and place it on a baking sheet, then pour the remaining fat in the pan over it.
12. Cook the stuffed heart in the oven for 16 to 22 min.
13. Once the time is up, cover the stuffed heart with a piece of foil and let it rest for 12 min, then serve it and enjoy.

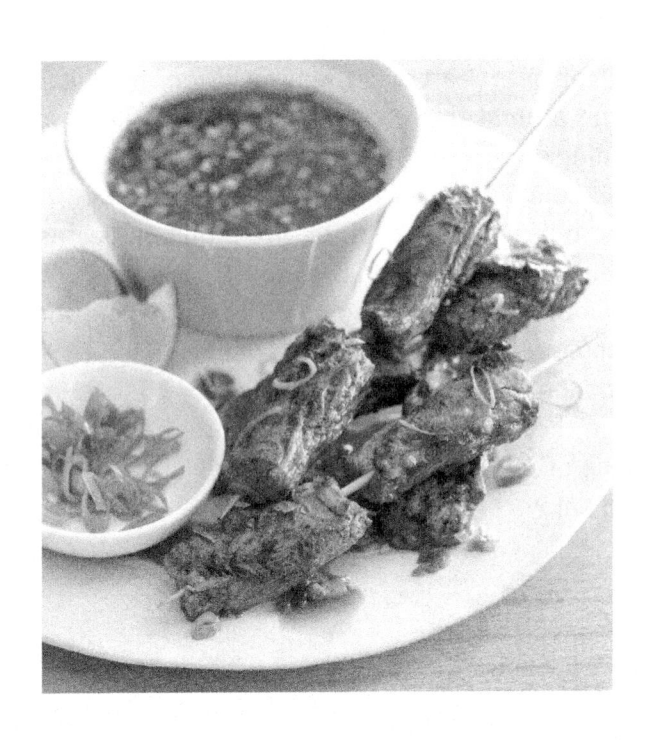

Orangy Steak Kebab

(Prep Time: 10 min | Cooking Time: 10 min | Servings 2 to 4)

Ingredients:

- 1 pound of lean beef, diced

- ¼ cup of fresh lime juice
- 2 tablespoons of coconut oil
- 1 small bunch of basil, leaves, finely chopped
- 1 teaspoon of orange zest, grated
- 1 teaspoon of cumin
- Black pepper
- Salt

Directions:

1. Before you do anything else preheat the grill and grease it.
2. Season the steak cubes with some salt and pepper.
3. Combine the lime juice with basil, coconut oil, orange zest and cumin in a food processor and process them until they become smooth.
4. Place the steak dices in a large zip lock bag and pour the basil mix all over it, then seal it and shake it to coat.
5. Place the bag in the fridge and let it sit for at least 30 min.
6. Thread the steak dices into skewers, then grill them for 8 to 10 min while turning them every once in a while.
7. Serve your skewers warm and enjoy.

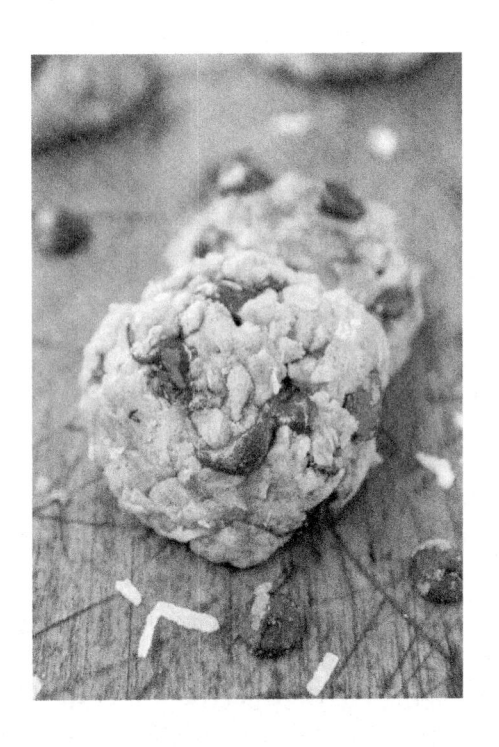

Chocolate Chip Cookies

(Prep Time: 10 min | Cooking Time: 13 min | Servings 12)

Ingredients:

- 1 ¼ cup of almond flour
- ½ cup of swerve sweetener, granulated
- 1/3 cup of low carb baking chocolate chips
- ¼ cup of butter
- 1 egg
- 3 tablespoons of coconut flour
- 15 drops of vanilla stevia
- 2 tablespoons of coconut oil
- 1 teaspoon of vanilla extract
- ½ teaspoon of baking soda
- Salt

Directions:

1. Before you do anything preheat the oven to 350 F.
2. Stir the almond flour with coconut flour, baking soda and a pinch of salt in a large mixing bowl.
3. Beat the butter with sweetener until they become smooth.
4. Add the egg with stevia, coconut oil, and vanilla extract, then beat them again until they become creamy.
5. Add the mix to the flour mix, then stir them until they are well combined.
6. Fold the baking chocolate chips into the batter, then spoon it with an ice cream spoon to a lined baking sheet to make 12 cookies.
7. Bake the chocolate chip cookies for 11 to 13 min, then serve them and enjoy.

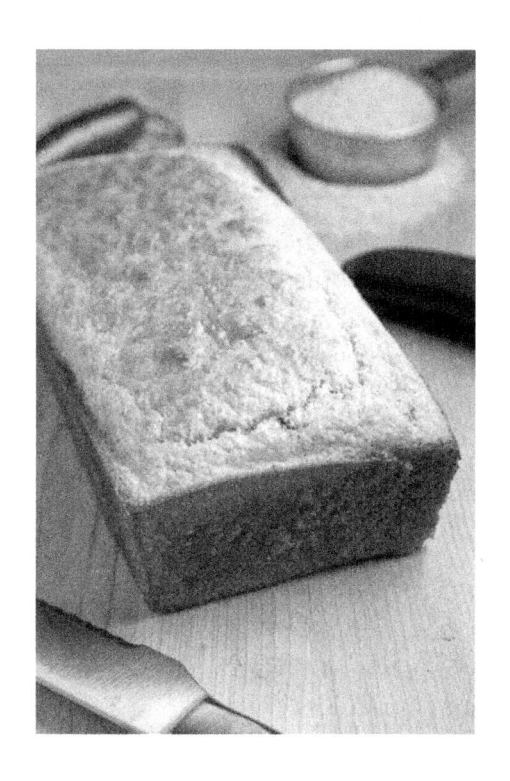

Cheesy Cornbread Bacon

(Prep Time: 10 min | Cooking Time: 22 min | Servings 8)

Ingredients:

- 2 cups of almond flour
- 5 eggs
- 1 cup of cheddar cheese, shredded
- 5 bacon sliced, cooked and crumbled
- ¼ cup of golden flax meal
- 2 tablespoons of apple cider vinegar
- ½ teaspoon of baking soda
- 1/8 teaspoon of corn extract
- Black pepper
- Salt

Directions:

1. Before you do anything preheat the oven to 350 F.
2. Whisk the eggs with vinegar and corn extract in a large mixing bowl until they become frothy.
3. Add the remaining ingredients with a pinch of salt, then whisk them until they become smooth.
4. Pour the batter into a greased pan and bake it in the oven for 22 min.
5. Once the time is up, serve your cheesy cornbread with your favorite toppings and enjoy.

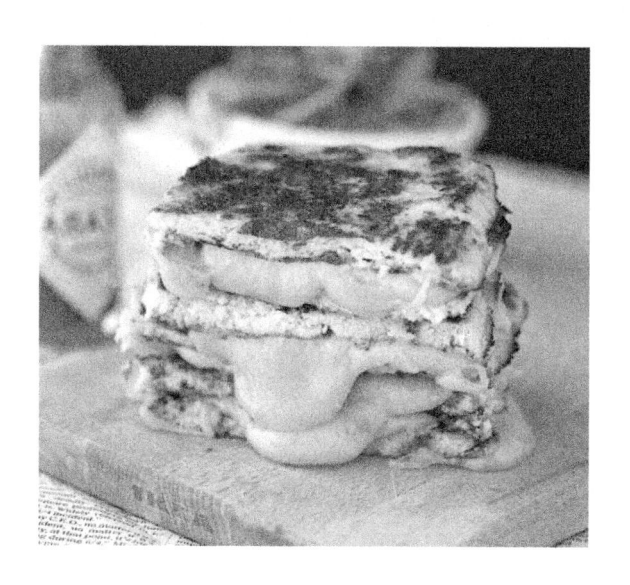

Melted Sandwich

(Prep Time: 15 min | Cooking Time: 20 min | Servings 4)

Ingredients:

- 1 medium head of cauliflower, chopped
- ½ cup of parmesan cheese, grated
- 1 egg
- 2 slices of cheddar cheese, thick

- 1 teaspoon of Italian seasoning
- Black pepper
- Salt

Directions:

1. Before you do anything preheat the oven to 450 F.
2. Place the chopped cauliflower in a food processor, then process it until it becomes like rice.
3. Pour the cauliflower rice into a microwave safe bowl, then microwave it for 2 min.
4. Stir the cauliflower, then microwave it for 3 min.
5. Stir the cauliflower again and microwave it for 5 min, then repeat the process once again.
6. Place the cauliflower bowl aside and let it sit for 6 min to lose heat.
7. Add the parmesan cheese with Italian seasoning, egg, a pinch of salt and pepper to the cauliflower and mix them well.
8. Divide the mix into 4 portions, then shape them into a square bread slices, then place them on a lined-up baking sheet.
9. Cook the cauliflower slices in the oven for 16 to 19 min, then place them aside to cool down for few minutes.
10. Preheat the oven broiler.

11. Place a cheese slice on top of 2 cauliflower slices, then cover them with the other 2 slices and bake them in the oven broiler for 4 to 6 min.

12. Serve your cheesy cauliflower sandwiches and enjoy.

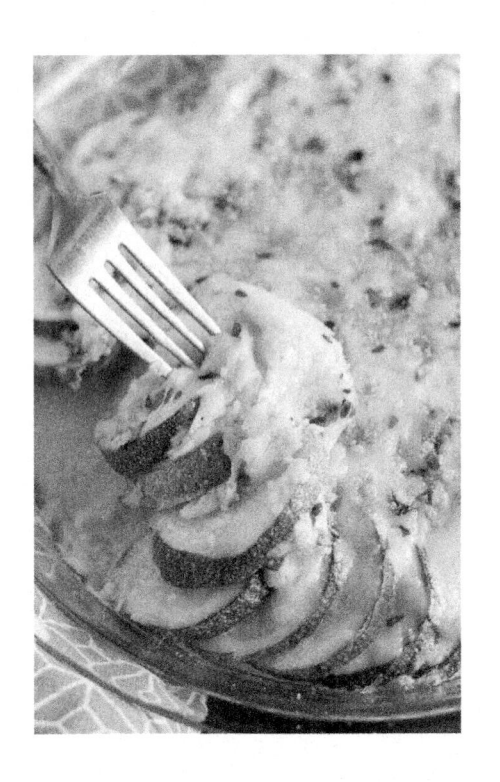

Golden Cheese Gratin

(Prep Time: 10 min | Cooking Time: 47 min | Servings 6)

Ingredients:

4 cups of fresh zucchini, sliced
1 ½ cup of pepper jack cheese, shredded
1 small yellow onion, peeled and thinly sliced
½ cup of heavy whipping cream
2 tablespoons of butter
½ teaspoon of garlic powder
Black pepper
Salt

Directions:

- Before you do anything preheat the oven to 375 F.
- Lay 1/3 of the zucchini slices in the bottom of a greased baking dish, then top it with 1/3 of the onion, a pinch of pepper, a pinch of salt and ½ cup of cheese.
- Repeat the process to create 2 more layers.
- Mix the whipping cream with butter, garlic powder and a pinch of salt in a small microwave safe bowl, then microwave them for 1 min.
- Pour the mix all over the zucchini casserole, then bake it for 47 min.
- Once the time is up, serve it warm and enjoy.

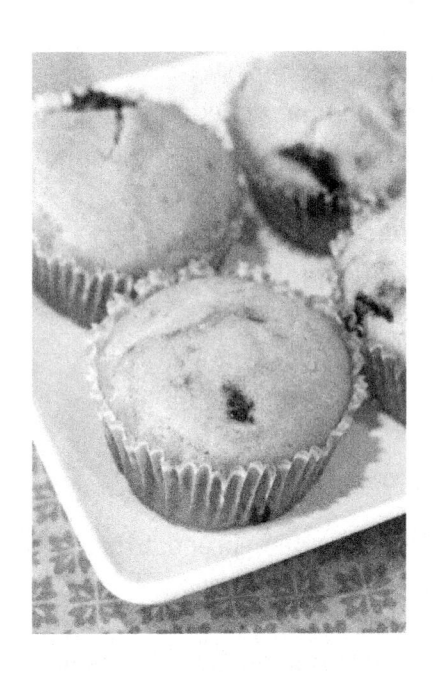

Spring Muffins

(Prep Time: 15 min | Cooking Time: 32 min | Servings 6)

Ingredients:

- ½ cup of coconut flour
- 1/3 cup of fresh blueberries

- ¼ cup and 2 teaspoons of swerve sweetener, granulated
- ¼ cup of heavy cream
- 3 eggs
- 2 ounces of butter, soft
- 4 tablespoons of cream cheese
- 1 teaspoon of baking powder
- ½ teaspoon of vanilla extract
- 1/8 teaspoon of xanthan gum, ground
- Salt

Directions:

1. Before you do anything preheat the oven to 350 F.
2. Stir the coconut flour with xanthan gum, baking powder and a pinch of salt in a large mixing bowl.
3. Beat the butter with cream cheese and vanilla extract in another mixing bowl until they become creamy.
4. Add 1/3 of the flour mix and beat them until they become smooth and light, then add the 1 egg and beat them again.
5. Repeat the process with the remaining flour and eggs while mixing the batter gently until it becomes light.
6. Add the heavy cream and whisk them until they become smooth and light, then fold the blueberries into the batter.

7. Pour the batter into 6 muffins lined up pan, then bake them for 6 min.
8. Lower the temperature to 350 F, then bake them for an extra 26 min.
9. Allow the muffins to cool down for a while, then serve them and enjoy.

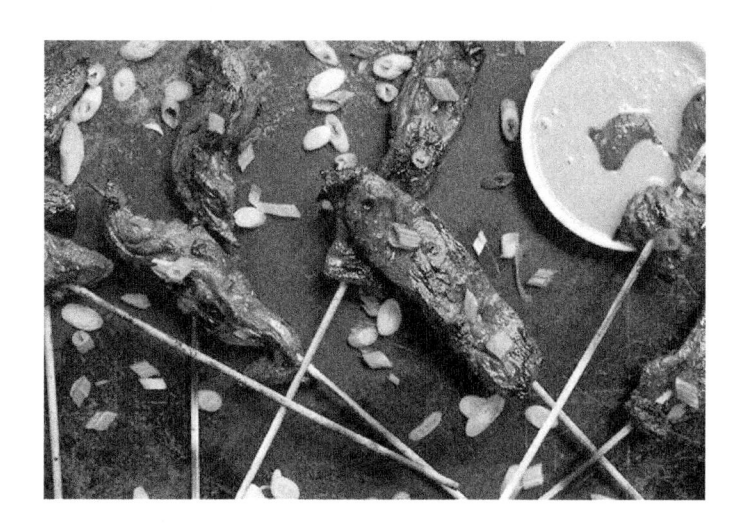

Tamari Steak Satay

(Prep Time: 10 min | Cooking Time: 12 min | Servings 4)

Ingredients:

- 1 pound of flank steak, cut into strips
- 2 tablespoons of tamari soy sauce
- 2 tablespoons of fish sauce
- 2 tablespoons of swerve sweetener, granulated

- 1 tablespoon of olive oil
- Black pepper
- Salt

Directions:

1. Season the flank steak strips with some salt and pepper.
2. Whisk the soy sauce with fish sauce and sweetener to make the marinade.
3. Pour the marinade all over the steak strips, then stir them to coat and place the bowl in the fridge for 20 to 30 min or more.
4. Once the time is up, preheat the grill and grease it.
5. Drain the steak strips from the marinade and thread them onto skewers, then brush them with olive oil.
6. Grill the steak strips for 3 to 6 min on each side or until they are done to your liking, then serve them warm and enjoy.

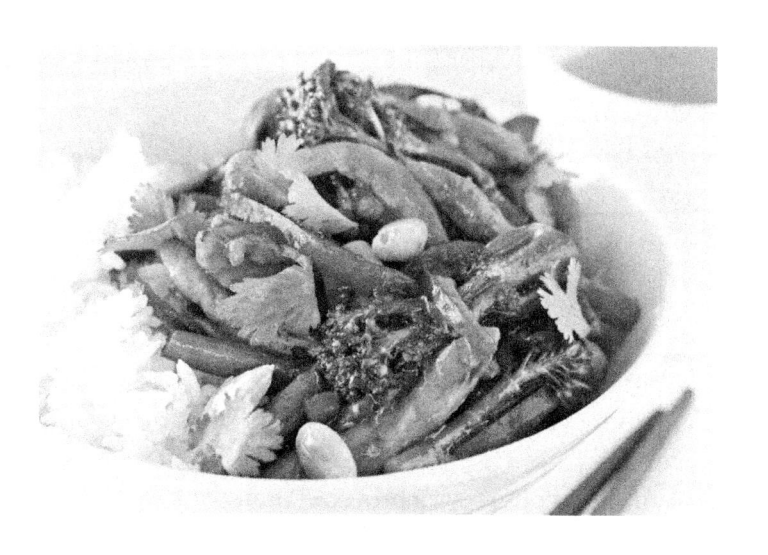

Meaty Rainbow Stir Fry

(Prep Time: 5 min | Cooking Time: 20 min | Servings 6)

Ingredients:

2 pounds of pork shoulder, sliced
12 ounces of butter
5 bell peppers, thinly sliced
1 cup of broccoli florets
6 tablespoons of almonds

- 1 tablespoon of swerve sweetener, granulated
- 3 teaspoons of chili paste
- Black pepper
- Salt

Directions:

1. Melt the butter in a large pan or a wok, then brown the pork strips until they become golden brown and cooked.
2. Add the peppers with broccoli, then cook them for 5 min while stirring often.
3. Add the chili paste with sweetener, almonds, a pinch of salt and pepper, then cook them for 1 to 2 min.
4. Serve your stew warm and enjoy.

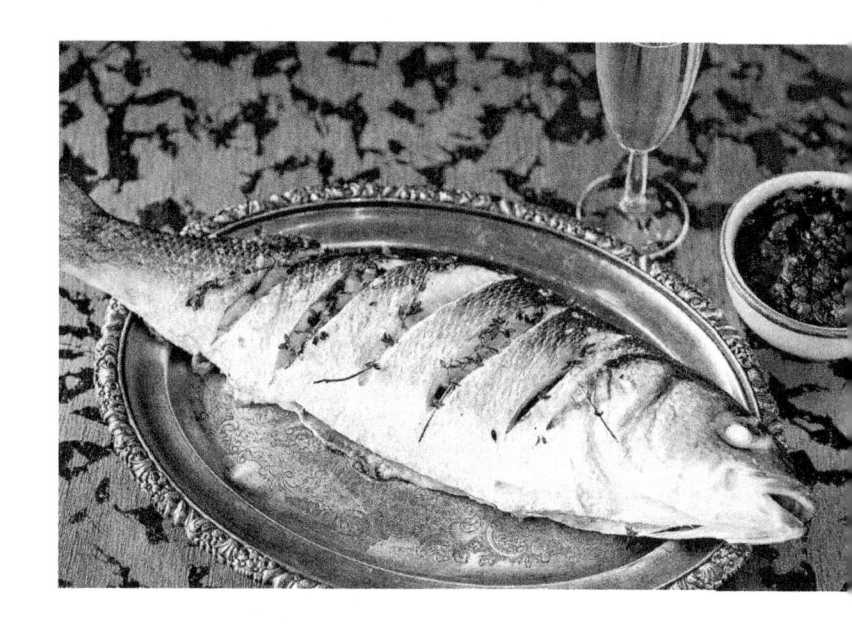

Minty Wild Sea Bass

(Prep Time: 5 min | Cooking Time: 16 min | Servings 2)

***

Ingredients:

- 1 whole sea bass, 10 to 12 ounces
- ½ cup of parsley
- 2 small lemons, sliced

- 3 tablespoons of coconut oil, melted
- Black pepper
- Salt

Directions:

1. Before you do anything preheat the oven to 400 F.
2. Place the lemon slices with parsley inside the fish, then place on a baking sheet.
3. Season the fish with some salt and pepper, then pour the coconut oil over it.
4. Use a sharp knife to create several slits on the side facing up of the fish, then bake it for 16 min.
5. Serve your baked sea bass warm and enjoy.

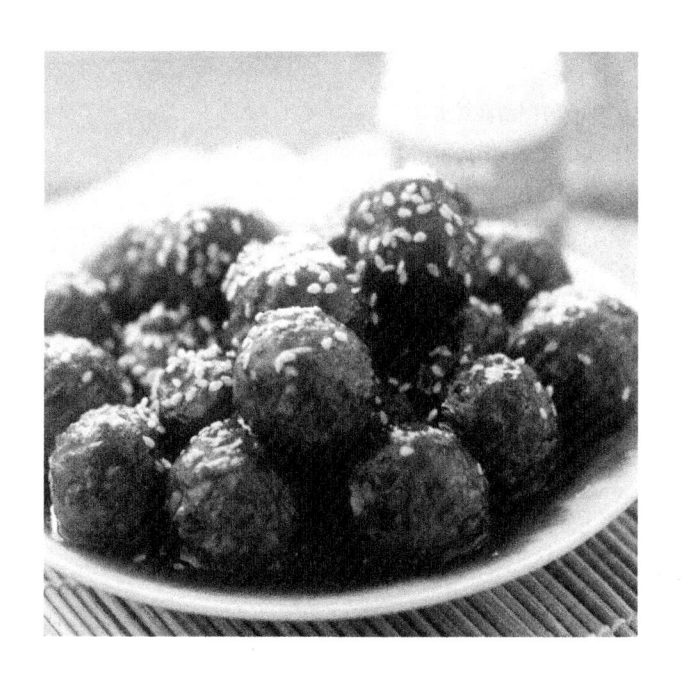

Sweet and Sour Apple Meatballs

(Prep Time: 10 min | Cooking Time: 20 min | Servings 4)

Ingredients:

- 1 pound of lean beef, minced
- 1 ½ cup of water

- 1 cup of erythritol
- 1/3 cup of ketchup, sugar free
- ¼ cup of parmesan cheese, grated
- ¼ cup of apple cider vinegar
- 1 egg
- 3 tablespoons of soy sauce
- ½ teaspoon of onion powder
- ½ teaspoon of xanthan gum, ground
- Black pepper
- Salt

Directions:

1. Combine the beef with onion powder, cheese, egg, some salt and pepper in a large mixing bowl, then mix them well with your hands.
2. Shape the mix into bite size meatballs.
3. Heat a greased skillet over medium heat, then brown in it the meatballs until they become golden brown.
4. Drain the meatballs and place them aside.
5. Stir the water with erythritol in the same pan until it dissolves.
6. Add the ketchup with soy sauce, vinegar and a pinch of salt, then cook them over medium heat while whisking all the time until the sauce starts boiling.
7. Add the xanthan gum and stir it, then lower the heat and simmer the sauce until it thickens slightly.

- Add the meatballs to the sauce and cook them for 12 min over low heat.
- Once the time is up, serve your saucy meatballs warm and enjoy.

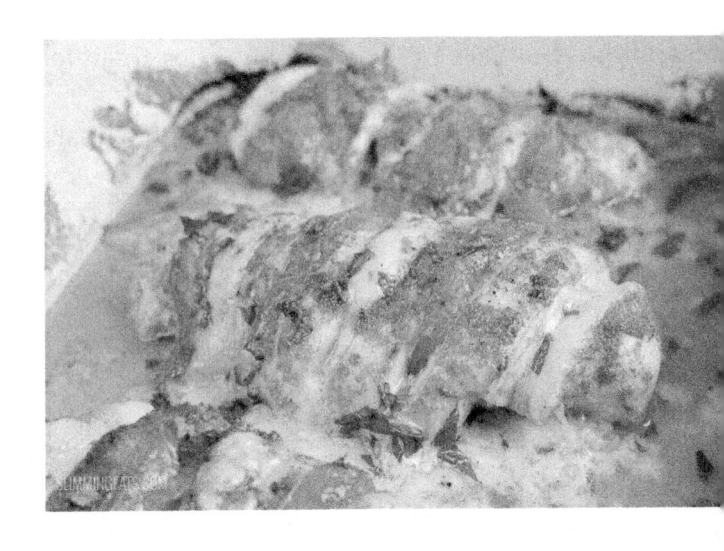

Grammy Hassel-back Chicken Winner

(Prep Time: 10 min | Cooking Time: 28 min | Servings 6)

Ingredients:

- 3 chicken breasts halved
- 18 mozzarella slices
- 18 tomato slices
- ¼ cup of chicken broth
- 1 tablespoon of olive oil

- Black pepper
- Salt

Directions:

1. Before you do anything preheat the oven to 400 F.
2. Use a sharp knife to make 6 slices in each chicken breast half without cutting it all the way through.
3. Season the chicken breasts with some salt and pepper, then place them in a baking dish.
4. Stuff 1 slit of each chicken breast halve with 1 slice of cheese and another one with 1 slice of tomato, then keep alternating between them.
5. Pour the broth on the side of the chicken breasts and drizzle the olive oil over the stuffed chicken breasts.
6. Baked the stuffed chicken breasts for 26 to 28 min or until they are done, then serve them warm and enjoy.

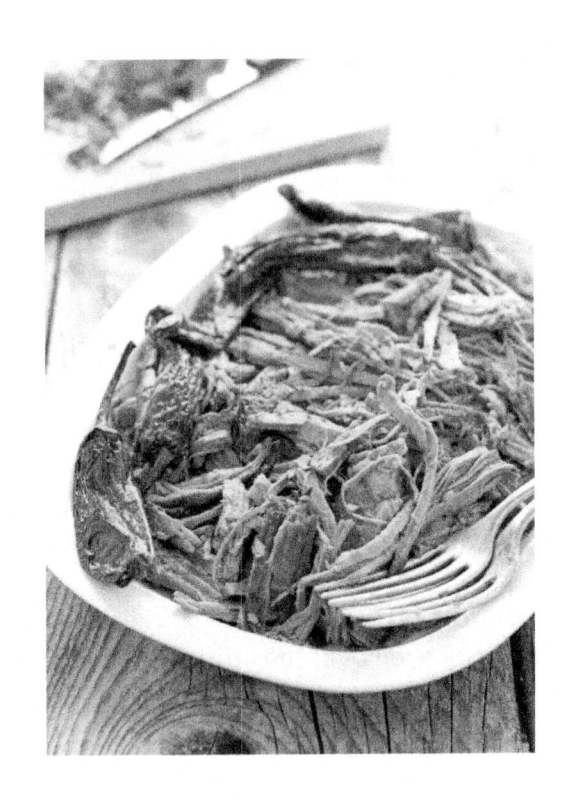

Shredded River Roast

(Prep Time: 15 min | Cooking Time: 10 h | Servings 8 to 10)

Ingredients:

- 4 pounds chuck roast, cut into pieces
- 16 ounces of canned pepperoni pepper, drained and sliced
- ½ cup of butter
- 1 tablespoon of dry drill
- 1 tablespoon of garlic powder
- 1 tablespoon of onion powder
- 1 tablespoon of dry parsley
- Black pepper
- Salt

Directions:

1. Place the chuck roast pieces in a slow cooker, then top them with the remaining ingredients.
2. Put on the lid and cook them for 9 to 10 h.
3. Once the time is up, drain the roast pieces and shred them with a fork, then stir them back into the pot.
4. Serve your shredded river roast warm and enjoy.

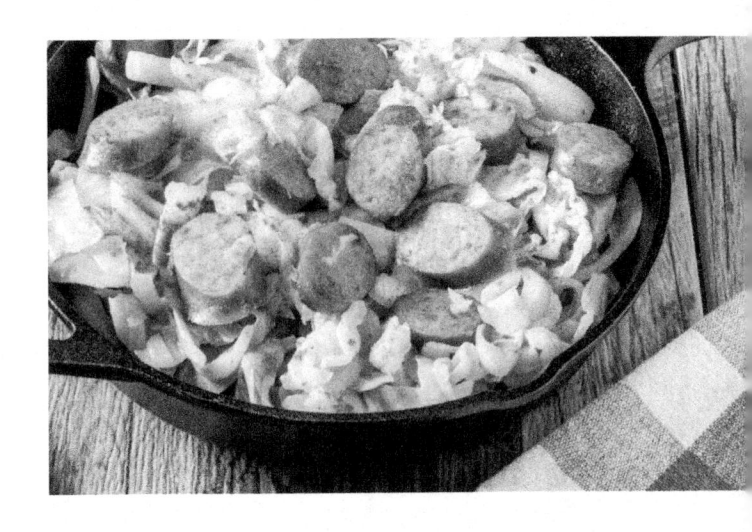

Tasty Lunch Rush Skillet

(Prep Time: 10 min | Cooking Time: 20 min | Servings 4)

Ingredients:

- 4 Italian chicken sausages, sliced
- 3 cups of cabbage, thinly sliced
- ½ cup of onion, diced
- 2 Colby Jack cheese slices
- 2 tablespoons of coconut oil

- Black pepper
- Salt

Directions:

1. Melt the coconut oil in a large skillet, then sauté in it the onion with cabbage for 9 min.
2. Add the chicken sausages and cook them for another 9 min while stirring them often.
3. Place the cheese slices on top, then put on the lid and cook them for 1 to 3 min or until the cheese melts.
4. Serve your skillet warm and enjoy.

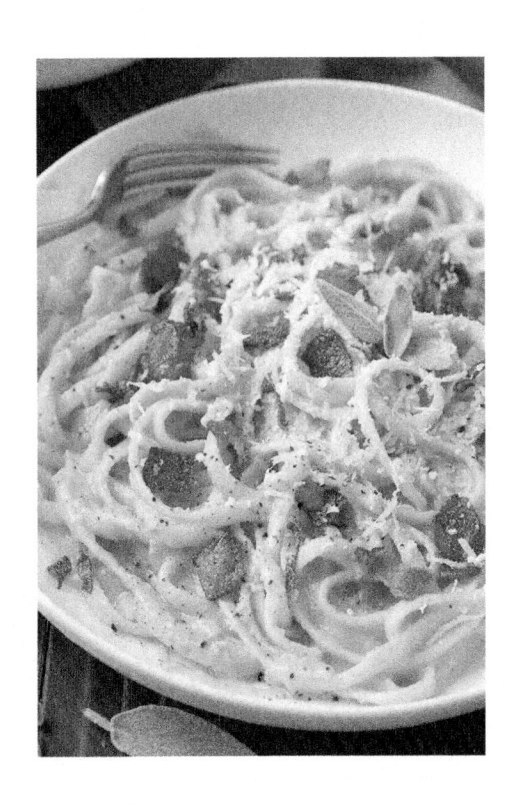

Creamy Bacon Carbonara

(Prep Time: 10 min | Cooking Time: 20 min | Servings 3)

Ingredients:

- 1 package of shirataki noodles
- 5 ounces of bacon, diced
- 1/3 cup of parmesan cheese, grated
- ¼ cup of heavy cream
- 2 egg yolks
- 3 tablespoons of pumpkin purée
- 2 tablespoons of butter
- ½ teaspoon of dry sage
- Black pepper
- Salt

Directions:

1. Cover the noodles with some hot water and let it sit for 3 min, then drain it and pat it dry.
2. Melt the butter in a saucepan and add to it the pumpkin purée with egg yolks and stir them well.
3. Add the heavy cream next.
4. Cook the bacon in a large skillet until it becomes crisp, then drain it and place it aside.
5. Add the noodles to the skillet with the bacon grease, then cook it for 5 min while stirring from time to time.
6. Stir the cheese into the sauce until it completely melts and cook the sauce until it becomes slightly thick.
7. Add the noodles to the sauce and stir it to coat, then serve it with the crisp bacon bits and enjoy.

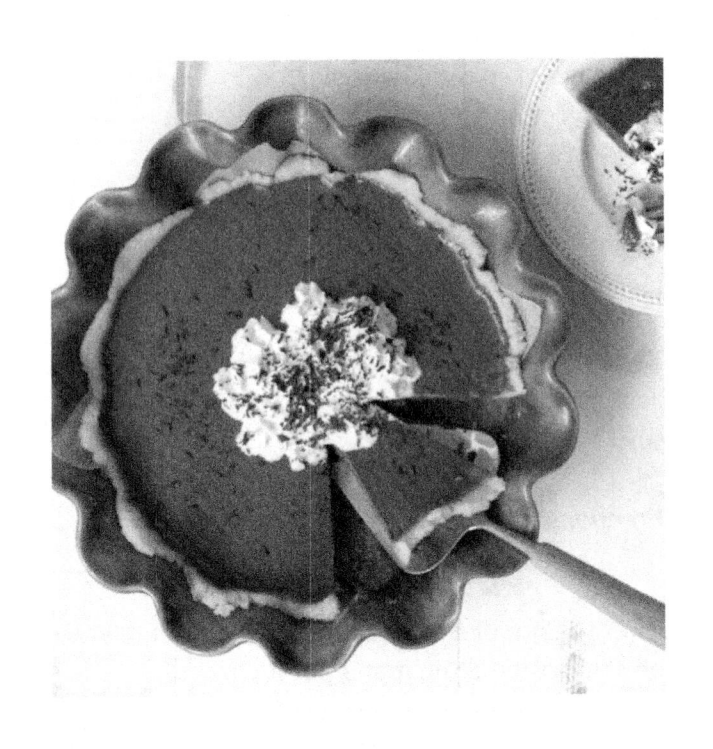

Love on a Plate

(Prep Time: 15 min | Cooking Time: 14 min | Servings 10)

Ingredients:

- 16 ounces of cream cheese
- 1 ½ cup of almond flour
- 1 cup of whipping cream
- ½ cup and 1/3 cup of erythritol, powdered
- ½ cup of cocoa powder
- 1 egg
- 7 tablespoons of butter
- 4 tablespoons of sour cream
- 2 ½ teaspoons of vanilla extract
- 2 teaspoon of erythritol, granulated
- ½ teaspoon of baking powder
- Salt

Directions:

1. Before you do anything preheat the oven to 375 F.
2. Stir the baking powder with 1/3 cup of erythritol, and a pinch of salt in a large mixing bowl.
3. Add 3 tablespoons of butter to the flour mix and mix them well with your hands.
4. Add 1 ½ teaspoon of vanilla extract to the flour mix, then mix them well until you get a soft dough.
5. Roll the dough on a lightly floured surface, then transfer it to a greased baking pan and cut off the edges.

6. Prick the dough several times with a fork, then bake it in the oven for 14 min until it becomes golden.

7. Beat 4 tablespoons of butter with cream cheese, sour cream, ½ cup of erythritol, and cocoa powder in a large mixing bowl until they become creamy.

8. Beat the whipping cream in another mixing bowl until it soft peaks.

9. Add 1 teaspoon of vanilla extract and the granulated erythritol, then beat it again until it becomes smooth.

10. Spoon 1/3 of the whipped cream to the chocolate cream mix and fold it gently, then add the remaining whipped cream and combine them well.

11. Spoon the mix into the pie shell after it completely cools down, then chill it in the fridge until ready to serve and enjoy.

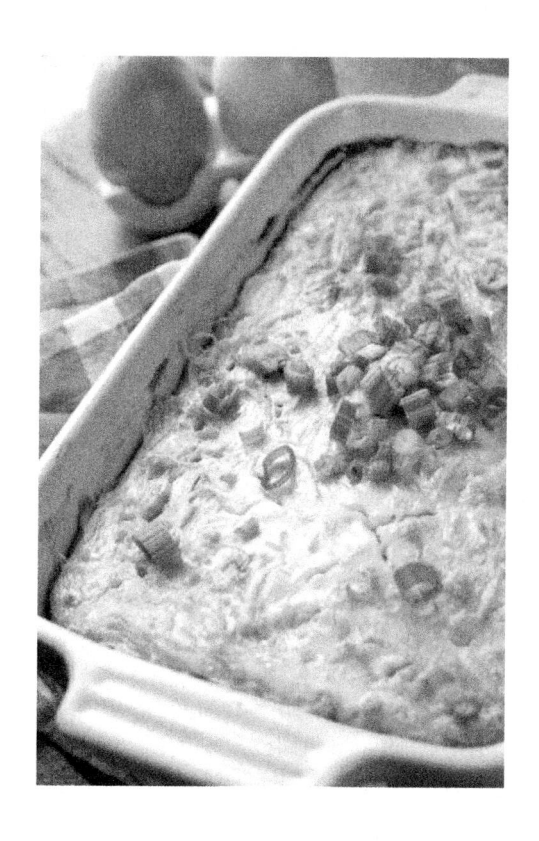

Frank's Hot Buffalo Casserole

(Prep Time: 15 min | Cooking Time: 55 min | Servings 6)

Ingredients:

- 2 pounds of chicken thighs, boneless and skinless
- 12 ounces of cream cheese
- 4 ounces of cheddar cheese, shredded
- 2 ounces of mozzarella cheese, shredded
- 3 jalapenos, seeded and sliced
- 6 bacon slices, diced
- ¼ cup of mayonnaise
- ¼ cup of Frank's red hot sauce
- Black pepper
- Salt

Directions:

1. Before you do anything preheat the oven to 400 F.
2. Season the chicken thighs with some salt and pepper.
3. Line a baking sheet with a piece of foil and place a cooling rack over it.
4. Place the chicken thighs on top, then bake them for 42 min.
5. Cook the bacon in a large skillet until it becomes crisp.
6. Add the jalapenos and cook them for 3 min.
7. Stir the hot sauce with mayonnaise and cream cheese until they are well combined, then turn off the heat.

8. Place the chicken thighs in a greased casserole dish, then top it with the sauce mix followed by the cheese.
9. Cook the buffalo chicken casserole in the oven for 13 to 17 min, then serve it warm and enjoy.

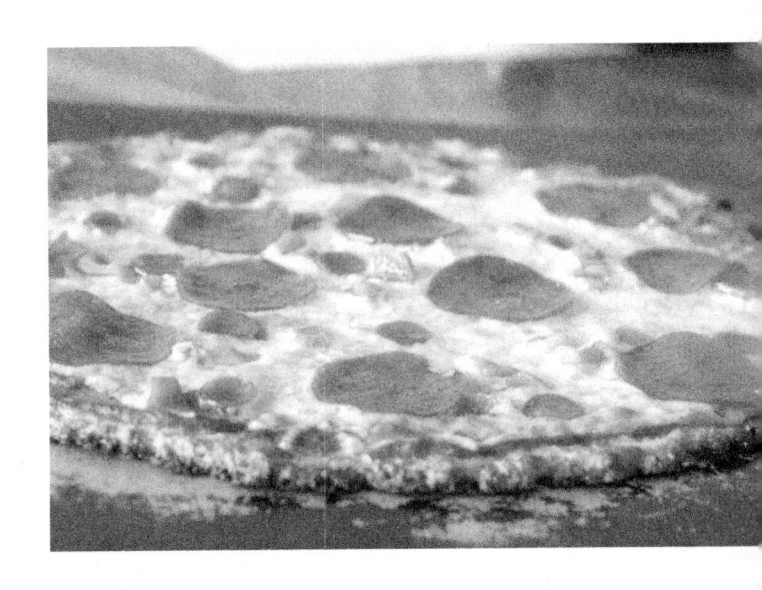

Italian Style Pepperoni Pizza

(Prep Time: 10 min | Cooking Time: 24 min | Servings 6)

Ingredients:

- 3 cups of mozzarella cheese, shredded
- ¾ cup of almond flour
- ½ cup of tomato sauce
- 16 pepperoni slices

- 3 tablespoons of cream cheese
- 1 egg
- 1 tablespoon of psyllium husk powder
- 1 tablespoon of Italian seasoning
- Black pepper
- Salt

Directions:

1. Before you do anything preheat the oven to 400 F.
2. Place 2 cups of mozzarella cheese in a microwave safe bowl, then microwave it for 90 sec.
3. Add the cream cheese right away to the melted cheese with the egg and mix them well.
4. Add the almond flour with psyllium husk powder, Italian seasoning, a pinch of salt and pepper, then mix them well again until you get a smooth dough.
5. Knead the dough with your hands until it becomes soft, then roll it on a lightly floured surface into a round shape.
6. Transfer the pizza crust to a lined-up baking sheet, then bake it for 11 min.
7. Turn the pizza crust to the other side and cook it for an extra 3 to 5 min.
8. Sprinkle 1 cup of mozzarella cheese over the crust, then top it with the pepperoni slices.
9. Cook the pizza in the oven for 4 to 6 min, then serve it warm and enjoy.

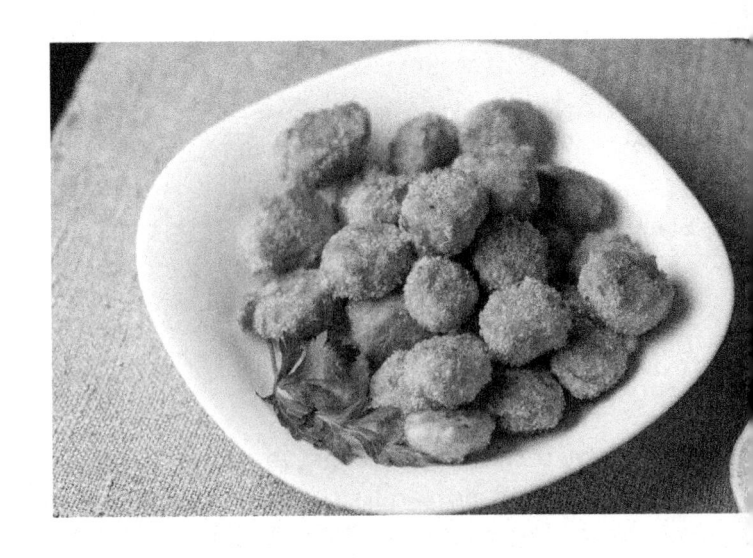

Nutty Chicken Bites

(Prep Time: 10 min | Cooking Time: 8 min | Servings 16)

Ingredients:

- 1 pound of lean chicken, minced
- 1 cup of almond flour
- 1 egg
- 1 egg, beaten
- 2 tablespoons of oil

2 tablespoons of coconut flour
½ teaspoon of paprika
½ teaspoon of onion powder
¼ teaspoon of rosemary, minced
1/8 teaspoon of garlic powder
Black pepper
Salt

Directions:

- Mix the chicken with ½ cup of almond flour, 1 egg, ¼ teaspoon of paprika, onion and garlic powder, a pinch of salt and pepper in a large mixing bowl with your hands.
- Shape the mix into bite-size meatballs and flatten them a bit with your hands.
- Mix the coconut flour with ¼ teaspoon of paprika, ½ cup of almond flour and a pinch of salt in a shallow bowl.
- Dip the chicken balls in the beaten egg, then coat them with the flour mix.
- Heat the oil in a large skillet, then cook in it the chicken balls for 2 to 4 min on each side until they become golden brown.
- Serve your chicken bites with your favorite sauce and enjoy.

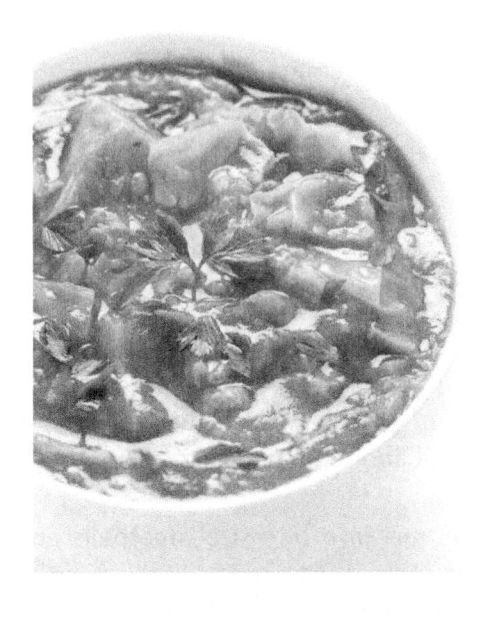

Chicken Rolls Soup

(Prep Time: 10 min | Cooking Time: 1 h 12 min | Servings 8)

Ingredients:

- 2 pounds of lean chicken, minced
- 16 ounces of marinara sauce
- 8 cups of cabbage, sliced
- 5 cups of chicken broth
- 2 cups of cauliflower, riced
- ½ cup of white onion, finely chopped
- ½ cup of shallot, finely chopped
- 2 tablespoons of olive oil
- 2 cloves of garlic, minced
- ½ teaspoon of dry oregano
- Black pepper
- Salt

Directions:

1. Heat the oil in a large soup pot, then sauté in it the garlic with onion with shallot for 6 min.
2. Add the chicken with oregano and cook them for another 6 min.
3. Stir the remaining ingredients into the pot, then put on the lid and cook them for 1 h over low heat.
4. Serve your chicken rolls soup warm and enjoy.

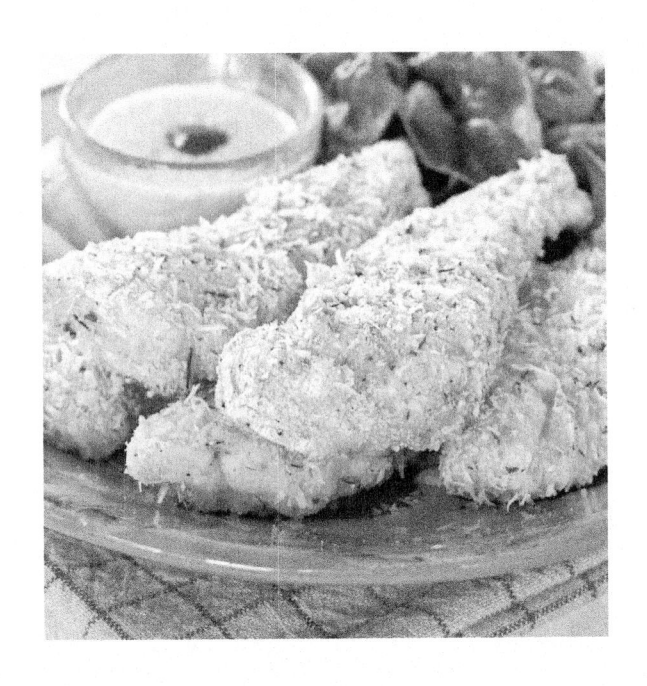

Crispy Parmesan Nuggets

(Prep Time: 10 min | Cooking Time: 32 min | Servings 8)

Ingredients:

- 2 ½ pounds of chicken tenderloins
- 1 1/8 cup of parmesan cheese, grated

- ¾ cup of butter
- 1 teaspoon of garlic powder
- Black pepper
- Salt

Directions:

1. Before you do anything preheat the oven to 325 F.
2. Place the butter in a large pan, then melt the butter completely.
3. Stir in the garlic powder with cheese until they melt.
4. Dip the chicken tenders in the melted butter mix, then place them on a lined-up baking sheet.
5. Cook the chicken tenders in the oven for 28 to 32 min or until they become golden brown.
6. Serve your chicken tenders with your favorite dip and enjoy.

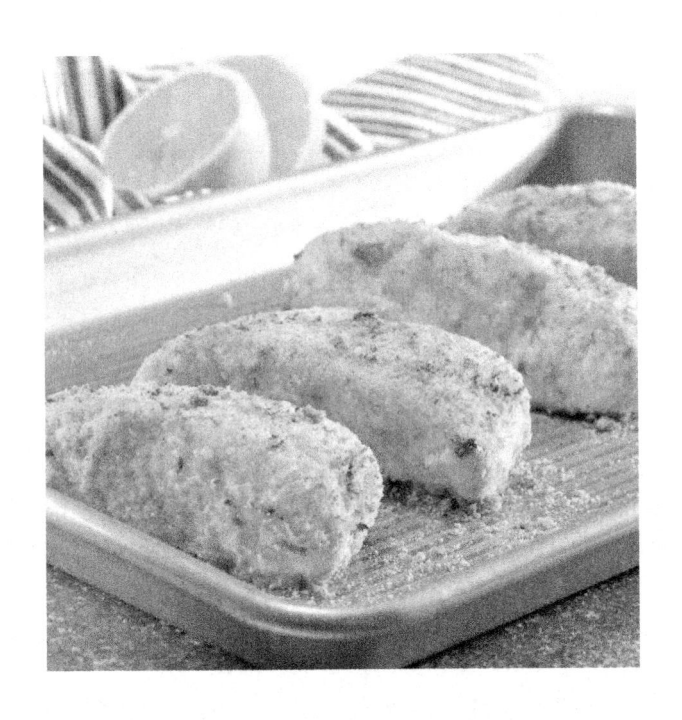

Parmesan Sea Knight

(Prep Time: 10 min | Cooking Time: 14 min | Servings 4 to 6)

Ingredients:

- 2 pounds of halibut fillets

¾ cup of butter, melted
¼ cup of parmesan cheese, grated
2 tablespoons of panko breadcrumbs
1 tablespoon of dry parsley
2 teaspoons of garlic powder
Black pepper
Salt

Directions:

- Before you do anything preheat the oven to 400 F.
- Sliced the halibut fillets into pieces, then season them with some salt and pepper.
- Whisk the cheese with melted butter, breadcrumbs, parsley, garlic powder, a pinch of salt and pepper in a mixing bowl.
- Dip the halibut pieces in the batter and coat them with it, then place them on a lined baking sheet.
- Bake the crusted halibut in the oven for 12 to 14 min or until it becomes golden, then serve it warm and enjoy.

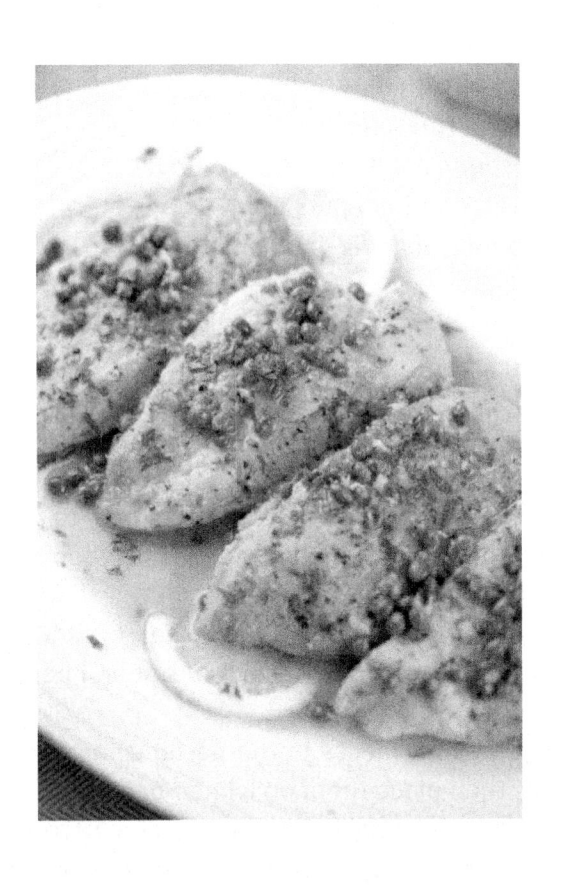

Tipsy Chicken Picatta

(Prep Time: 10 min | Cooking Time: 24 min | Servings 6)

Ingredients:

- 4 chicken breasts, skinless
- ¾ cup of butter
- ½ cup of chicken stock
- ¼ cup of heavy cream
- ¼ cup of olive oil
- ¼ cup of white wine
- ¼ cup of brined capers
- ¼ cup of fresh lemon juice
- ¼ cup of parsley, finely chopped
- Black pepper
- Salt

Directions:

1. Season the chicken breasts with some salt and pepper.
2. Melt 2 tablespoons of butter with olive oil in a large skillet, then cook the chicken breasts for 6 to 8 min on each side or until they become golden brown.
3. Drain the chicken breasts and place them aside.
4. Stir the white wine into the skillet and cook it until it reduces by half.
5. Stir the capers with lemon juice and stock, then cook them until they start boiling.

6. Add the chicken breasts to the pan and cook them for an extra 5 min.

7. Drain the chicken breasts and place them aside.

8. Add the cream with remaining butter, a pinch of salt and pepper to the sauce in the pan, then whisk them until the sauce becomes slightly thick.

9. Pour the sauce all over the chicken breasts, then serve them warm and enjoy.

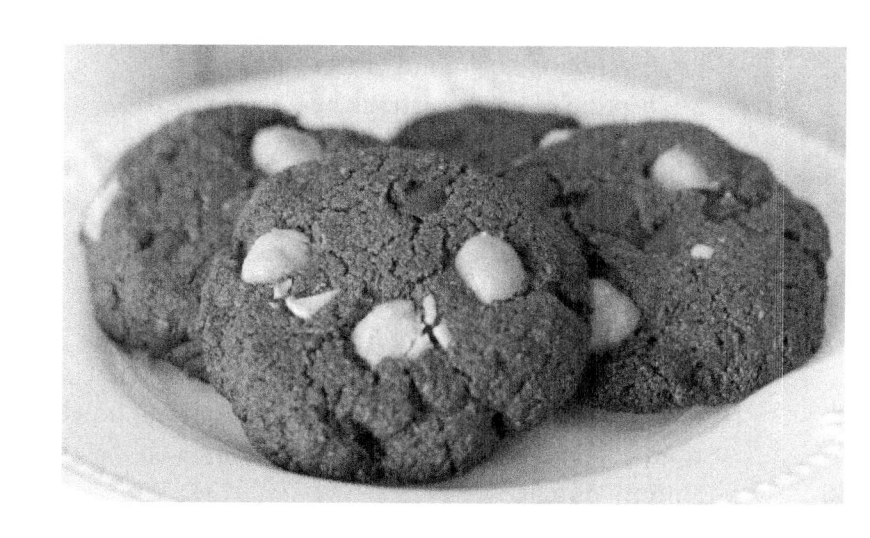

Macadamia Snap Cookies

(Prep Time: 10 min | Cooking Time: 16 min | Servings 16)

Ingredients:

- 1 ½ cup of almond flour
- ½ cup of erythritol, powdered
- ½ cup of butter, melted
- ¼ cup of macadamia nuts, roughly chopped
- 1 egg

- 2 tablespoons of almond butter
- 1 teaspoon of vanilla extract
- ½ teaspoon of baking soda
- Salt

Directions:

1. Before you do anything preheat the oven to 350 F.
2. Combine all the ingredients in a large mixing bowl, then mix them with your hands until you get a smooth dough.
3. Shape the mix into 1 ½ inch balls and flatten them slightly, then place them on a lined-up baking sheet.
4. Cook the cookies in the oven for 16 min.
5. Once the time is up, allow the cookies to cool down completely, then serve them and enjoy.

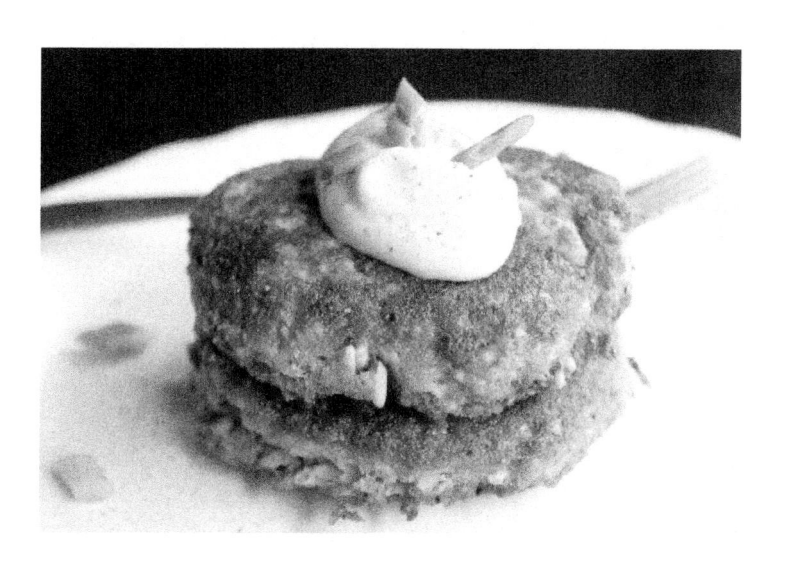

Salmon fritters

(Prep Time: 8 min | Cooking Time: 10 min | Servings 4)

Ingredients:

14 ounces of canned pink salmon, drained
2 ounces of salmon, smoked and chopped
1/3 cup of almond flour
1 egg

- 3 tablespoons of ranch dressing
- 2 tablespoons of parsley, finely chopped
- 2 tablespoons of avocado oil
- 1 teaspoon of Cajun seasoning
- Black pepper
- Salt

Directions:

1. Whisk the ranch dressing with egg in a large mixing bowl.
2. Add the canned and smoked salmon with flour, parsley, Cajun seasoning, some salt and pepper, then mix them well.
3. Shape the mix into medium sized 8 patties.
4. Heat the avocado oil in a large skillet, then cook the patties until they become golden brown on each side.
5. Serve your patties with your favorite toppings and enjoy.

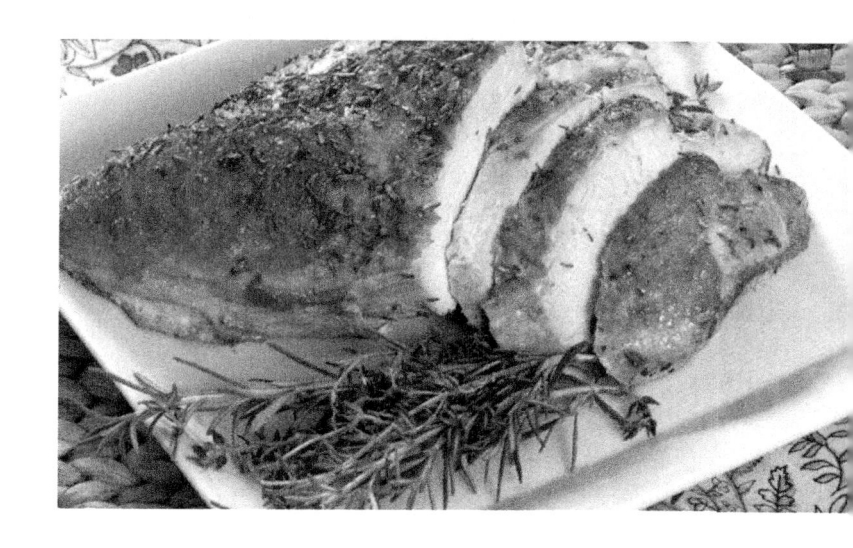

Festive Turkey Breast Roast

(Prep Time: 12 min | Cooking Time: 1 h 16 min | Servings 12 to 16)

Ingredients:

- 8 pounds turkey roast
- 1 cup of porcini mushroom, sliced
- ¼ cup of mayonnaise
- ¼ cup of butter, softened
- 1 tablespoon of turkey seasoning

- 1 tablespoon of rosemary, finely chopped
- Black pepper
- Salt

Directions:

1. Place the dry porcini in a food processor, then process it until it becomes powdered.
2. Add the turkey seasoning with a pinch of salt and pepper, then pulse them several times.
3. Whisk the butter with mayonnaise in a mixing bowl until they become creamy.
4. Add the mushroom mix with rosemary, then mix them again.
5. Season the turkey breast with some salt and pepper.
6. Before you do anything preheat the oven to 400 F.
7. Coat the turkey breast with the mushroom mix, then place it in the oven and cook it for 1 h 16 min.
8. Wrap the turkey breast with a piece of foil and place it aside to rest for 5 min, then serve it and enjoy.

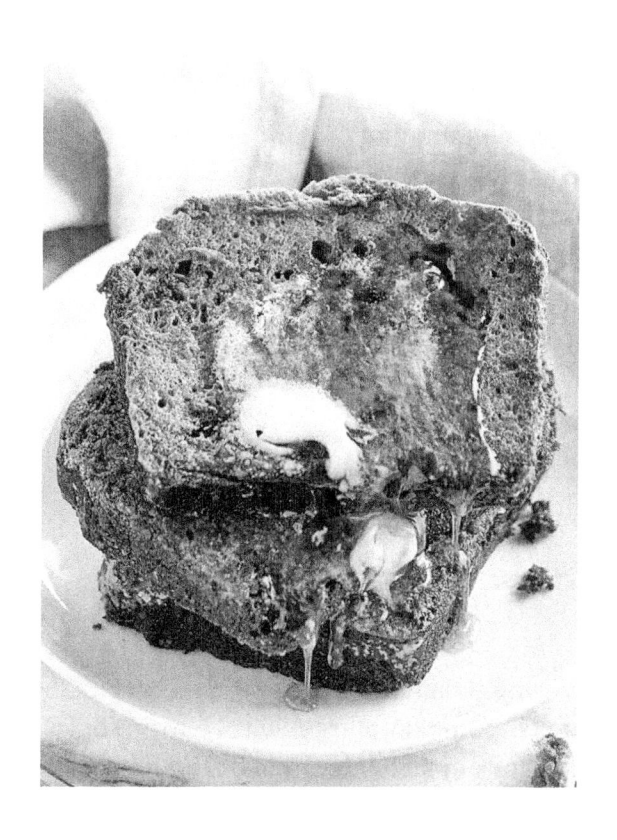

Tanned Pumpkin Toast

(Prep Time: 10 min | Cooking Time: 1 h | Servings 8 slices)

Ingredients:

- 2 cups of almond flour
- 1 cup of pumpkin purée
- ¾ cup of butter, melted
- 1/3 cup of coconut flour
- 4 eggs
- ¼ cup of almond milk
- 4 teaspoons of baking powder
- 1 teaspoon of cinnamon
- ¼ teaspoon of nutmeg powder
- Salt

Directions:

1. Before you do anything preheat the oven to 350 F.
2. Combine pumpkin purée with butter, eggs, and almond milk in a blender, then blend them smooth.
3. Stir the almond flour with coconut flour, baking powder, cinnamon, nutmeg powder and a pinch of salt in a large mixing bowl.
4. Add the egg mix, then whisk them until you get a smooth batter.
5. Pour the batter into a greased loaf pan, then bake it for 1 h.
6. Once the time is up, turn off the heat and allow the pumpkin bread to cool down completely.
7. Slice the pumpkin loaf, then prepare your toast the way you desire and enjoy.

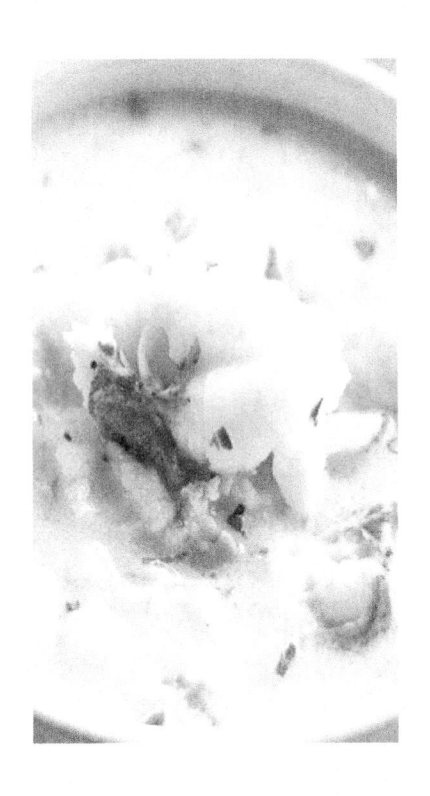

Restaurant Style Lobster Chowder

(Prep Time: 10 min | Cooking Time: 24 min | Servings 6)

Ingredients:

- 3 cups of almond milk
- 2 cups of lobster broth
- 2 cups of lobster, cooked
- 2 cups of cauliflower florets
- ½ cup of onion, finely chopped
- ¼ cup of butter
- 2 tablespoons of parsley, finely chopped
- 2 tablespoon of apple cider vinegar
- ¼ teaspoon of xanthan gum
- ¼ teaspoon of garlic powder
- Black pepper
- Salt

Directions:

1. Melt the butter in a large soup pot, then sauté the onion for 5 min.
2. Add cauliflower with broth, then put on the lid and cook them for 7 min.
3. Stir in the milk, then cook the soup for an extra 3 min.
4. Spoon some of the broth in a small bowl, then stir in the xanthan gum and pour it back into the pot.
5. Add the remaining ingredients to the pot and cook them for another 3 to 5 min.
6. Adjust the seasoning of the soup, then serve it warm and enjoy.

Conclusion

Thank you again for downloading this book! I really do hope you found these keto recipes as tasty and mouthwatering as I did, and if you've already reached this page, I'm sure the keto diet is working its magic as we speak. Best of luck to you and your friends and family with whom you share these delicious meals with. Weight loss is a step by step process, and you've already conquered the hardest one; taking action!

Printed in Great Britain
by Amazon